TURNING POINTS

By Therese Harasymiw

THE BLACK DEATH

Cavendish Square

New York

Published in 2022 by Cavendish Square Publishing, LLC, 29 E. 21st Street
New York, NY 10010

First Edition

Website: cavendishsq.com

Portions of this work were originally authored by Don Nardo and published as *The Black Death* (*World History*). All new material this edition authored by Therese Harasymiw.

All websites were available and accurate when this book was sent to press.

Library of Congress Cataloging-in-Publication Data

Names: Harasymiw, Therese, author.
Title: The Black Death / Therese Harasymiw.
Description: New York : Cavendish Square Publishing, [2022] | Series: Turning points | Includes bibliographical references and index.
Identifiers: LCCN 2020023265 | ISBN 9781502660787 (library binding) | ISBN 9781502660770 (paperback) | ISBN 9781502660794 (ebook)
Subjects: LCSH: Black Death—Juvenile literature. | COVID-19—Juvenile literature. | Epidemics—Juvenile literature.
Classification: LCC RC172 .H337 2022 | DDC 362.196/2414—dc23
LC record available at https://lccn.loc.gov/2020023265

Editor: Therese Shea
Copy Editor: Abby Young
Designer: Deanna Paternostro

CPSIA compliance information: Batch #CS22CSQ: For further information contact Cavendish Square Publishing LLC, New York, New York, at 1-877-980-4450.

Printed in the United States of America

TABLE OF CONTENTS

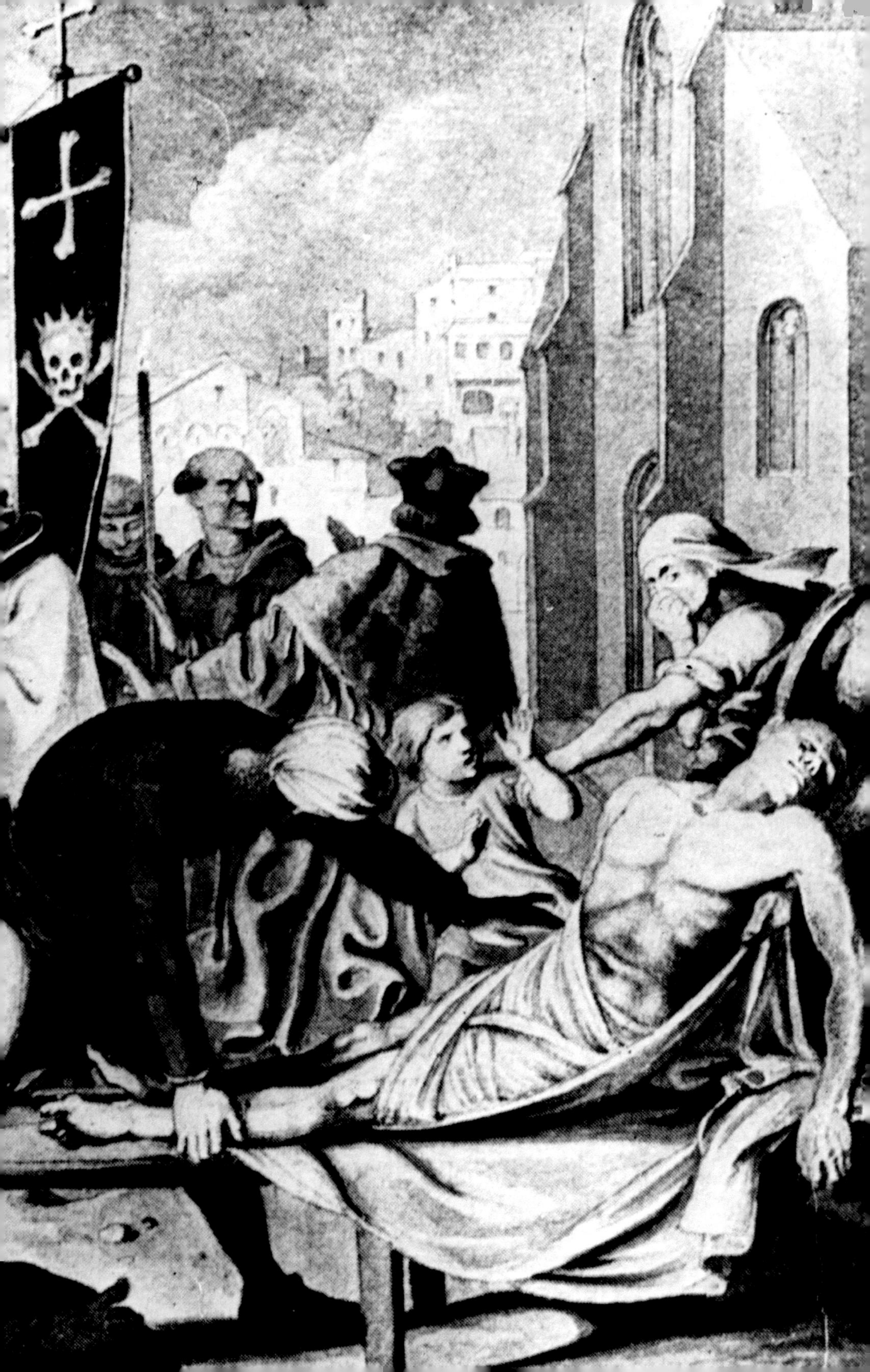

INTRODUCTION

A HORRIBLE CHAPTER IN HISTORY

In the beginning of his book *The Decameron*, Italian writer Giovanni Boccaccio provided a chilling glimpse of life in the middle of the 14th century in Florence, Italy:

> *Brothers abandoned each other, uncles abandoned their nephews, sisters abandoned their brothers, and wives frequently abandoned their husbands. And there is something else which is almost incredible: fathers and mothers were loath to visit and care for their children, almost as if they did not belong to them.*[1]

A terrible, life-altering event had struck Florence that tore apart not just society but families too. According to Boccaccio, even some parents ceased caring for their children. The regular relationships and routines of life had devolved into chaos. This turmoil was not just limited to Florence. It was infecting all of Europe and other parts of the world, as far east as Asia and as far south as North Africa. The cause of all this disorder? Plague.

Contagious Chaos

Plague is an infectious disease with deadly outcomes for humans if left untreated. In the 14th century, it was left untreated for an understandable reason: No one knew what it was. Countless people

Much art from the plague-ridden time of the Black Death depicts the misery of people, as they were constantly surrounded by death.

became extremely ill, experiencing great pain and often dying in a matter of days. The symptoms of the disease were frightening, especially when combined: fever, aching body parts, vomiting blood, and swollen glands in the neck, armpits, and groin called buboes. Buboes lend their name to the form of plague most historians think struck the world at this time—bubonic plague.

The disease could also cause the tissue around buboes and other parts of the body to die and turn black, giving the sickness the nickname the Black Death. (Some think the name came from the Latin term for the disease: *atra mors*. *Mors* means "death," and *atra* means "terrible" or "black.") Still other people called the disease the Great Pestilence.

While bubonic plague is the least deadly of the forms of plague, it wiped out millions of people across the communities it reached. Historians commonly debate the percentages, with 30 percent as the conservative estimate. That means three out of every ten people died in the parts of the world affected by the Black Death. Archaeological evidence, including mass graves, verifies corpses were piling up so rapidly that traditional individual burial was not possible. Whole cemeteries had to be created for victims of this plague.

Today, thanks to the work of a multitude of scientists, we know that the disease was caused by a bacterium. We even know the likely culprit for delivering the bacterium: fleas. However, at that time, the Black Death seemed supernatural. No one could understand how or why this undetectable enemy was spreading, and that led to the chaos described by Boccaccio. To many who hoped to survive, abandoning people infected by the disease—even loved ones—seemed the only course of action.

The Black Death's grip on the world lasted just a few years, and yet the world it touched was never the same after. Besides the millions of deaths, every aspect of life experienced altering shockwaves, including religion, art, education, society, and economics. Even the word "plague" became associated with more than just a specific disease. It has now come to mean any kind of deadly disease outbreak or event that causes widespread chaos and destruction.

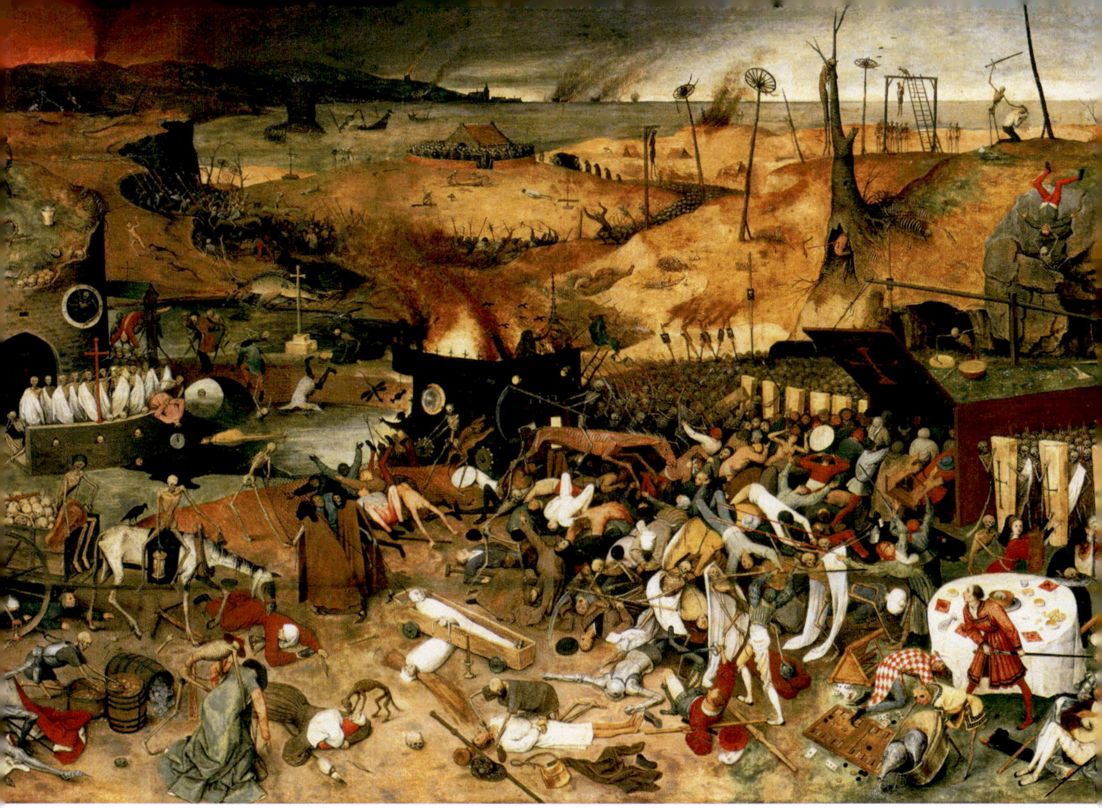

This painting from around 1562, called *The Triumph of Death*, demonstrates how the Black Death and plagues that followed made people feel that death was always near.

Historical Plagues

The people at the time of the Black Death felt they were experiencing the worst catastrophe in living memory. Boccaccio described it as, "So extraordinary that, if it had not been so often witnessed, and I had not seen it with my own eyes, I could scarcely believe it, let alone write about it."[7] Those who learn about the Black Death today often feel similarly. The high death toll, gruesome symptoms, and widespread destruction are so astonishing that in the age of modern medicine they are nearly unbelievable. The Black Death did cause such devastation, but it was not the first terrible plague the world experienced—and it would not be the last.

Historians often rely on written accounts, and sometimes those reports do not contain enough information to provide an accurate description of events. However, there are existing records of epidemics before the Black Death that may have been caused by plague.

The ancient Greek historian Thucydides wrote about a disease that struck the Greek city-state of Athens in 430 BCE. At the time, Athens was being attacked by the rival city-state Sparta. Athenians were taking refuge within the walls of their city when a mysterious illness struck with frightening speed. Thucydides explained:

> *People in perfect health suddenly began to have burning feelings in the head … Before long, the pain settled on the chest and was accompanied by coughing. Next the stomach was affected, with stomach-aches and with vomiting … The skin was rather reddish and livid, breaking out into small pustules [boils] and ulcers.*[3]

The sickness Thucydides described remains unidentified, but bubonic plague is one possibility. Whatever it was, it killed about 30 percent of Athens's residents, perhaps as many as 100,000 people.

More than 900 years later, a Byzantine historian named Procopius described the symptoms of a disease that struck Constantinople (present-day Istanbul, Turkey), a city in the Byzantine

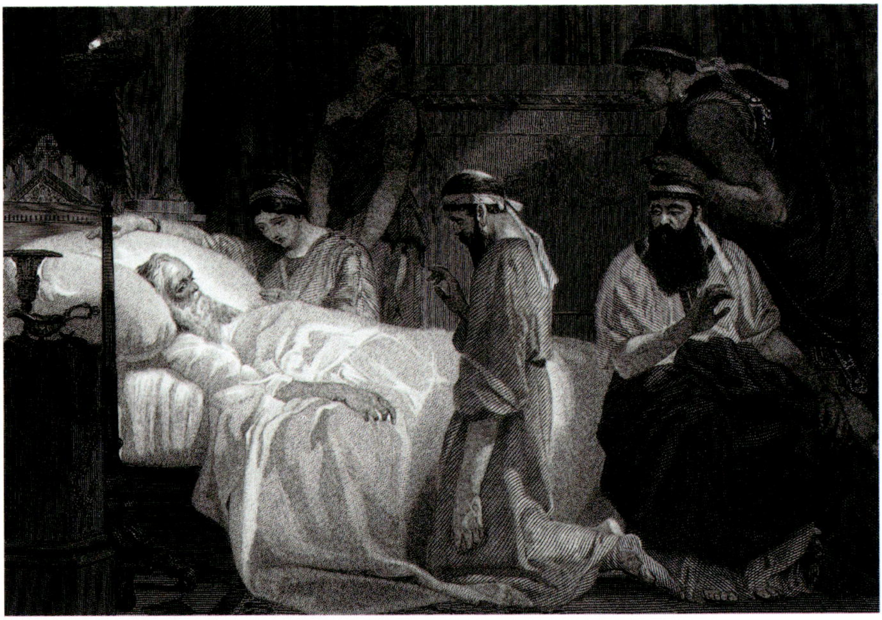

The plague that struck Athens infected a famous statesman named Pericles. His death in 429 BCE, disastrous for the city-state, is depicted in this engraving from 1870.

Empire, in 541 CE: "A bubonic swelling developed ... below the abdomen, but also inside the armpit, and in some cases also beside the ears, and at different points on the thighs."[4] It became known as Justinian's Plague, after the Byzantine emperor at the time, Justinian. The description of buboes and other details helped modern historians identify the infection as most likely bubonic plague. The plague spread into Europe and Asia. To Procopius, it seemed as if the deadly plague came close to eradicating the human race. In reality, scholars think about 20 to 40 percent of the people of Constantinople died, and perhaps around 25 percent of the Byzantine Empire, or more than 25 million people.

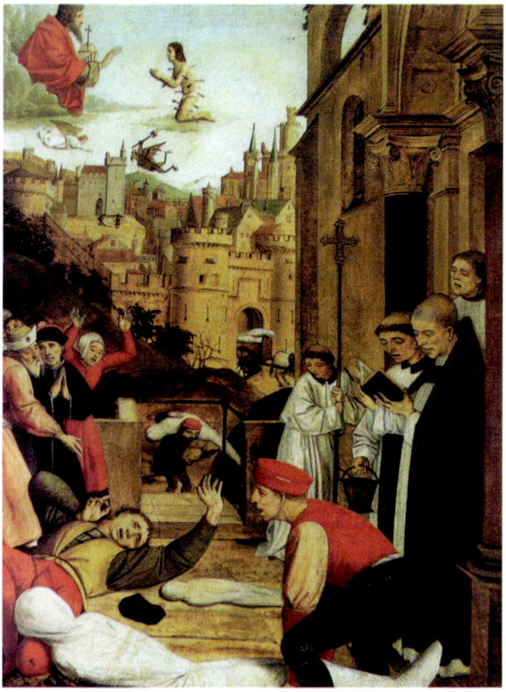

In this 15th-century painting depicting Justinian's Plague, a gravedigger falls victim to plague. St. Sebastian is shown in heaven, asking Jesus to heal the man.

Procopius noted that people could explain other kinds of diseases, but this disease was different: "It is quite impossible either to express in words or to conceive in thought any explanation, except indeed to [say the cause is] God."[5] This impression that the cause was something outside of humankind's control—perhaps something unearthly—was similar to how those who experienced the Black Death about 800 years later felt. Though other diseases, some quite deadly, were known to them, they had not seen anything like this plague, and the records of plagues that came before were not known or accessible to many back then as they are in the modern age. The world was helpless as tens of millions died of the Black Death.

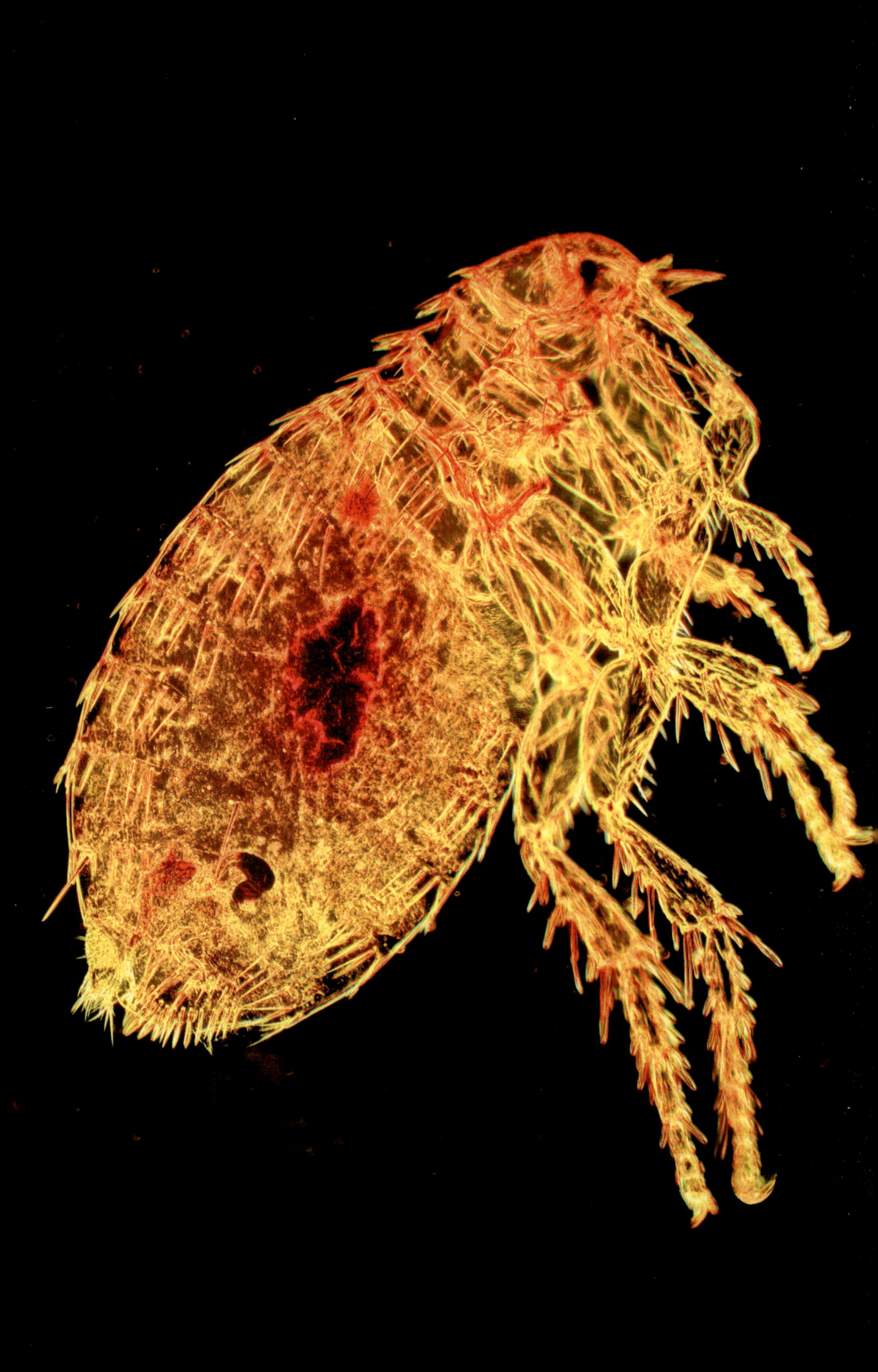

CHAPTER ONE

THE BLACK DEATH BEGINS

The Black Death of the 14th century was so devastating that it destroyed economies, communities, faiths, and even families. Few events in history have had such an impact as this plague. It became a pandemic, which means the outbreak affected a very high proportion of the population over a wide geographic area. Many historians point to two main reasons why it was so lethal: First, no one at the time knew what was spreading the illness. Second, without this knowledge, people did not know how to effectively slow the spread of or cure the disease.

For many centuries before the Black Death, Europeans had not experienced widespread disease. Most known diseases were not as contagious and affected only small groups of people. Malnutrition—a lack of healthy foods in the diet—caused many of the health problems that medieval people did have. A disease called Saint Anthony's fire (or ergotism) was a kind of poisoning caused by a fungus on rye and other grains. Leprosy, an infection that can badly damage the appearance of someone's face and limbs, was a concern, but it was not very infectious and rarely fatal. These diseases were known to Europeans. When the mysterious symptoms of the Black Death began to appear and victims began to multiply quickly, so did mass panic and hysteria.

In the 19th century, a scientist discovered the Oriental rat flea, shown here, could carry the plague bacterium and spread it by biting people.

People tried to escape areas with plague, unknowingly carrying it with them to other communities. As people fled and died, society broke down. To many, it seemed like the world was actually coming to an end. Certainly, the lives of those in affected regions would never be the same, even if they were the lucky ones to survive.

Its Origins

Although 14th-century Europeans did not know what caused the Black Death, they did have a good idea of where it came from. Several writers of the time, including the Italian Gabriel de Mussis, claimed that it entered Europe from "the East." To Europeans, "the East" was a general term for Asia, including the region now called the Middle East.

Modern experts confirm this assumption. Evidence has been found that suggests bubonic plague bacteria originated far to the east of Europe. One of the key clues was the 1885 discovery of an old graveyard near the ruins of a medieval Christian community by a large lake in south-central Asia named Issyk-Kul. To Europeans, this location would certainly be "the East." In the cemetery, a Russian archaeologist found an abnormally large number of graves that were dug in 1338 and 1339. Additionally, some of the grave markers said that the cause of death was some kind of disease.

Scientists believe that the disease reached the Issyk-Kul area from somewhere in central Asia, probably first spreading from animals to humans in that region. According to distinguished medical researcher Alfred J. Bollet, large rodents called marmots were trapped for their fur in central Asia and sold to traders around this time. Many of the marmots were found sick and dying by trappers, who still shipped their furs to buyers. Some of these furs contained fleas infected with plague, which then infected humans who received the furs.

From central Asia, modern experts estimate that the disease moved westward along the major trade routes leading to an area near the Black Sea. At the time, much of this western Asian region was ruled by the Mongols (called Tartars by medieval

PAST MEETS PRESENT: ZOONOTIC DISEASES

Zoonotic diseases are illnesses caused by germs that pass from animals to people. Animals can carry viruses, bacteria, parasites, and fungi that do harm to themselves and people. The animals may not seem sick, even when they are carrying germs that are dangerous to humans.

Zoonotic diseases are not uncommon. In fact, an estimated six out of every ten infectious diseases can be spread by animals either directly or indirectly, such as touching a surface or water an animal has touched, eating food that has been contaminated by an animal's germs, or by the bite of an insect. For example, it is widely accepted that fleas carried the Black Death plague bacterium and spread it by biting people.

Scientists estimate that 75 percent of new infectious diseases come from animals. In 2019, an infectious virus called COVID-19 emerged in China and spread around the world. The source of the virus is very likely animals as it is much like similar viruses carried by bats. However, the exact source of the first animal-to-human transmission of COVID-19 is not yet known.

Europeans). By the mid-1340s, many Mongols and others in the area had died of plague. The next area to be infected was Crimea, a highly populated peninsula to the north of the Black Sea.

There, in the winter of 1345 to 1346, a Mongol leader was attempting to capture the town of Kaffa. Located between the borders of Asia and Europe, Kaffa was a colony of Italian city-state Genoa and one of Europe's great trading centers. The Mongols, however, soon had more to deal with than capturing the town. According to Gabriel de Mussis, "The whole army was affected by a disease which overran the Tartars and killed thousands upon thousands every day." He added, "All medical advice and attention was useless; the Tartars died as soon as the signs of disease appeared on their bodies."[1] The Mongol leader saw what the unknown ailment was doing to his own soldiers and came up with a plan. Today, what he did is referred to as biological warfare. He ordered his army to use catapults to throw infected corpses into the city. Though the Genoese tried to dispose of the bodies quickly, plague soon spread among them.

Invading Europe

Between the Mongolian siege and the increasing sickness, many people were dying inside the town of Kaffa. Those who were still living were desperate to escape. Some did manage to board ships and sail southward into the Black Sea, but they did not realize that they were carrying this deadly disease with them. They brought plague first to Constantinople, the mighty Byzantine metropolis on the sea's southern shore. From the dock areas, the disease quickly spread into the city's streets. No neighborhood or building—small or large, rich or poor—was immune. By mid-1347, plague in Constantinople was an epidemic.

However, much worse was to come. Constantinople was a busy hub for traders from across the Mediterranean-European sphere. Traders and merchants came from all over Europe and Asia to sell their goods in the Byzantine city. When the traders and merchants left, their ships were carrying the disease. This caused the Black Death to move southward into the Mediterranean, bound for ports in Palestine, Egypt, North Africa, Greece, Italy, and beyond.

Italy was one of the first of these new regions to feel the deadly impact. In 1347, 12 vessels carried plague to the city of Messina in Sicily. Italian writer Michael of Piazza described the initial and crucial outbreak in Messina:

> *At the beginning of October … twelve Genoese galleys … entered the harbour of Messina. In their bones they bore so virulent [potent] a disease that anyone who only spoke to them was seized by a mortal [lethal] illness and in no manner could evade death. The infection spread to everyone who had any intercourse [contact] with the diseased [people] … Not only all those who had*

FROM THE SOURCE: MICHAEL OF PIAZZA'S ACCOUNT

Italian friar Michael of Piazza wrote about the terrifying spread of plague through the Italian city of Messina in 1347 and the effect it had on society:

> *Soon men hated each other so much that, if a son was attacked by the disease, his father would not tend him. If, in spite of all, he dared to approach him, he was immediately infected and could by no means escape death, but was bound to expire [die] within three days. Nor was this all: all those belonging to him, dwelling in the same house with him, even the cats and other domestic animals, followed him in death. As the number of deaths increased in Messina many desired to confess their sins to the priests and to draw up their last will and testament. But ecclesiastics [clergy], lawyers and attorneys refused to enter the houses of the diseased … Soon the corpses were lying forsaken in the houses. No ecclesiastic, no son, no father and no relation dared to enter, but they paid hired servants with high wages to bury the dead.*[1]

1. Quoted in Johannes Nohl, *The Black Death: A Chronicle of the Plague* (Yardley, PA: Westholme Publishing, 2006), pp. 18–19.

> *intercourse with them died, but also those who had touched or used any of their things. When the inhabitants of Messina discovered that this sudden death emanated [came] from the Genoese ships they hurriedly expulsed [ordered] them from their harbour and town. But the evil remained with them and caused a fearful outbreak of death.*[2]

From Europe's trading ports, the Black Death moved northward. In Italy, it struck all urban areas, including Padua, Pisa, Rome, and Florence, with a fury. Michael of Piazza described some of the frightening symptoms:

> *Those infected felt themselves penetrated by a pain throughout their whole bodies and, so to say, undermined. Then there developed on their thighs or on their upper arms a boil about the size of a lentil which the people called "burn boil" … This infected the whole body, and penetrated it so that the patient violently vomited blood. This vomiting of blood continued without intermission [stopping] for three days, there being no means of healing it, and then the patient expired [died].*[3]

Horrifying Effects

There were so many victims of the Black Death in each town that the streets were soon full of corpses. Boccaccio's *The Decameron* offers a look into the horror of the Black Death in Florence, Italy. Many people "finished up [their lives] on the streets," he wrote, and "those who did die in their homes, only made their neighbours aware of their death by the stench from their corrupted [decomposing] bodies." He continued:

> *The city was full of corpses. Most of them were dealt with in the same way by their neighbours, influenced as much by fear of being infected by the rotting bodies as by charity towards the dead. By themselves, or with the aid of bearers … they dragged the newly dead out of their homes and placed them upon their doorsteps, where anyone who passed by, particularly in the morning, could see countless numbers of them.*[4]

Having dead bodies piled up throughout a city was a problem, and Florence was not unique in this regard. Many other European cities began to see their dead pile up. What made this worse was another dilemma—the corpses needed to be removed, but no one wanted to touch them. People feared they might catch plague through bodily contact or even through being near the corpses at all. As a result, very few were willing to take on the

THEY MADE HISTORY: GIOVANNI BOCCACCIO

Italian author Giovanni Boccaccio lived from 1313 to 1375. Growing up, he was interested in literature, but his father wanted him to be a businessman. While studying in the Italian city of Naples, he fell in love with a woman he called La Fiammetta (from the Italian word *fiamma*, meaning "flame"). No one knows her real name, but he wrote about his love for her in some of his early works.

In 1340, Boccaccio moved to Florence and studied Greek and Roman writings. It was in this city that he wrote his most renowned work, *The Decameron*, likely between 1348 and 1353. This book is about 10 people who left Florence in 1348 because of the arrival of the Black Death. As they travel, they tell each other 100 tales in all. In his introduction to *The Decameron*, Boccaccio talks in detail about the plague's impact. His descriptions are used by historians today to understand more about the Black Death and its effects on society.

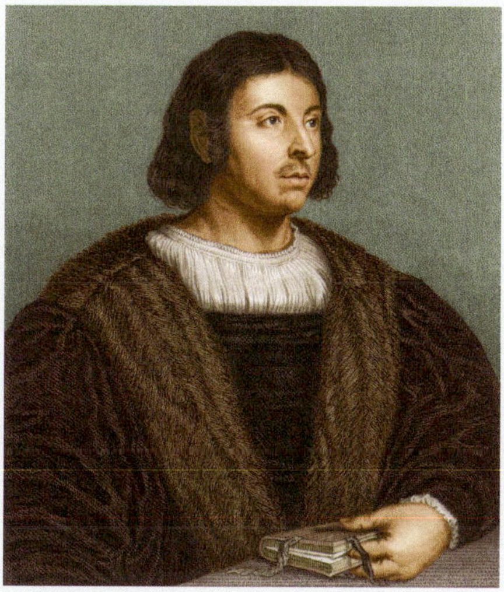

Giovanni Boccaccio was a humanist, which means he placed great importance on people, their capabilities, and their values.

awful task of burying the dead. In many cases, people ended up paying thugs and criminals to do it.

Still another problem with the masses of infected dead bodies was where to bury them. Most Europeans were Christians and expected to be buried in sacred ground, generally preferring cemeteries next to churches. As Boccaccio wrote:

> *There was not enough consecrated [sacred] ground to bury the great multitude of corpses arriving at every church every day and almost every hour … So, when all the graves were occupied, very deep pits were dug in the churchyards, into which the new arrivals were put in their hundreds. As they were stowed there, one on top of another, like merchandise in the hold of a ship, each layer was covered with a little earth, until the pit was full.*[5]

Mass graves such as this were often called plague pits. However, in some European cities, the deceased were sometimes burned. This

This painting from the 19th century is based on Boccaccio's description of events in Florence, Italy, during the Black Death.

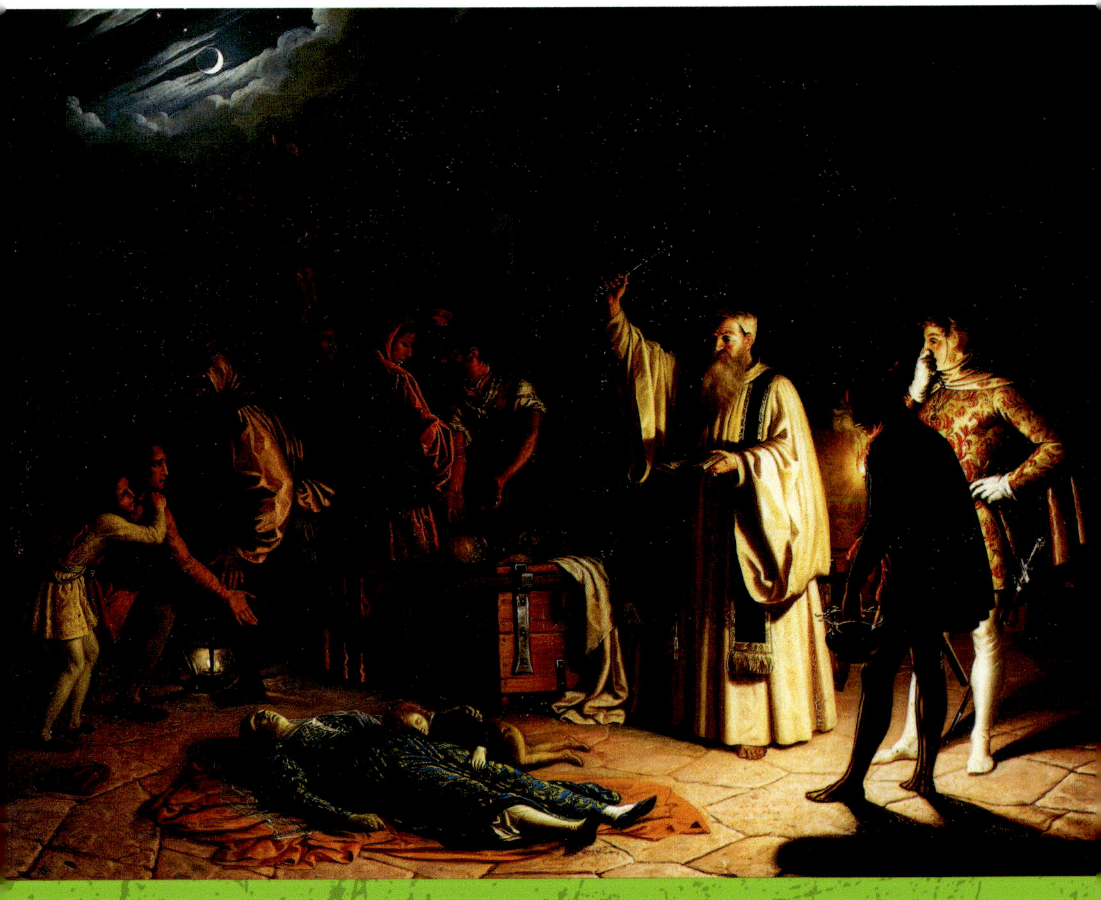

was done for two main reasons: There was not enough space, and fire was thought to cleanse infection. Land across Europe, especially land for cemeteries, was difficult to find. Although cremation had been a rare choice in medieval times, it was quickly adopted and used throughout Europe for thousands of corpses. In this way, not only were the streets cleared of bodies, but people also thought they were reducing their chances of being infected.

An intense fear of death overcame the population, Boccaccio observed. Because people believed they would probably die soon, they started behaving with no regard for the rules of society. Maintaining law and order in a diseased land was almost impossible.

Moving in All Directions

The epidemic spread northward into the heart of Europe, including the French city of Avignon, which was then the headquarters of the Catholic Church and Pope Clement VI. A leading member of the Church reported, to his horror, that half of Avignon's residents died in the outbreak's first two weeks alone.

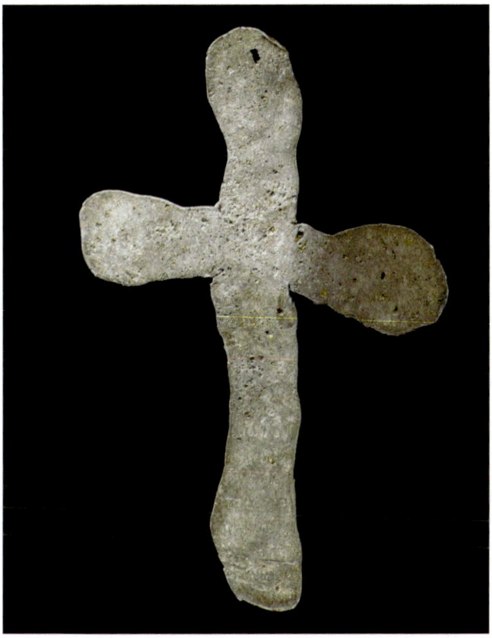

This lead cross was found on the body of a monk who died of plague in London, England. Many such crudely constructed crosses have been found on bodies recovered from that time.

After France had been devastated by the infection, the disease reached the banks of the English Channel. The English hoped that the wide waterway would protect them from the oncoming natural disaster. This, unfortunately, was not the case. Carried by the fleas on rats that stowed away on boats, the Black Death leapt across the channel. It spread from southern England northward, and less than a year after it arrived on England's shores, it reached the Scottish highlands and eastern Ireland.

Rats also stowed away on trading vessels headed to the lands today known as Germany, Poland, and Russia. The Russian city of

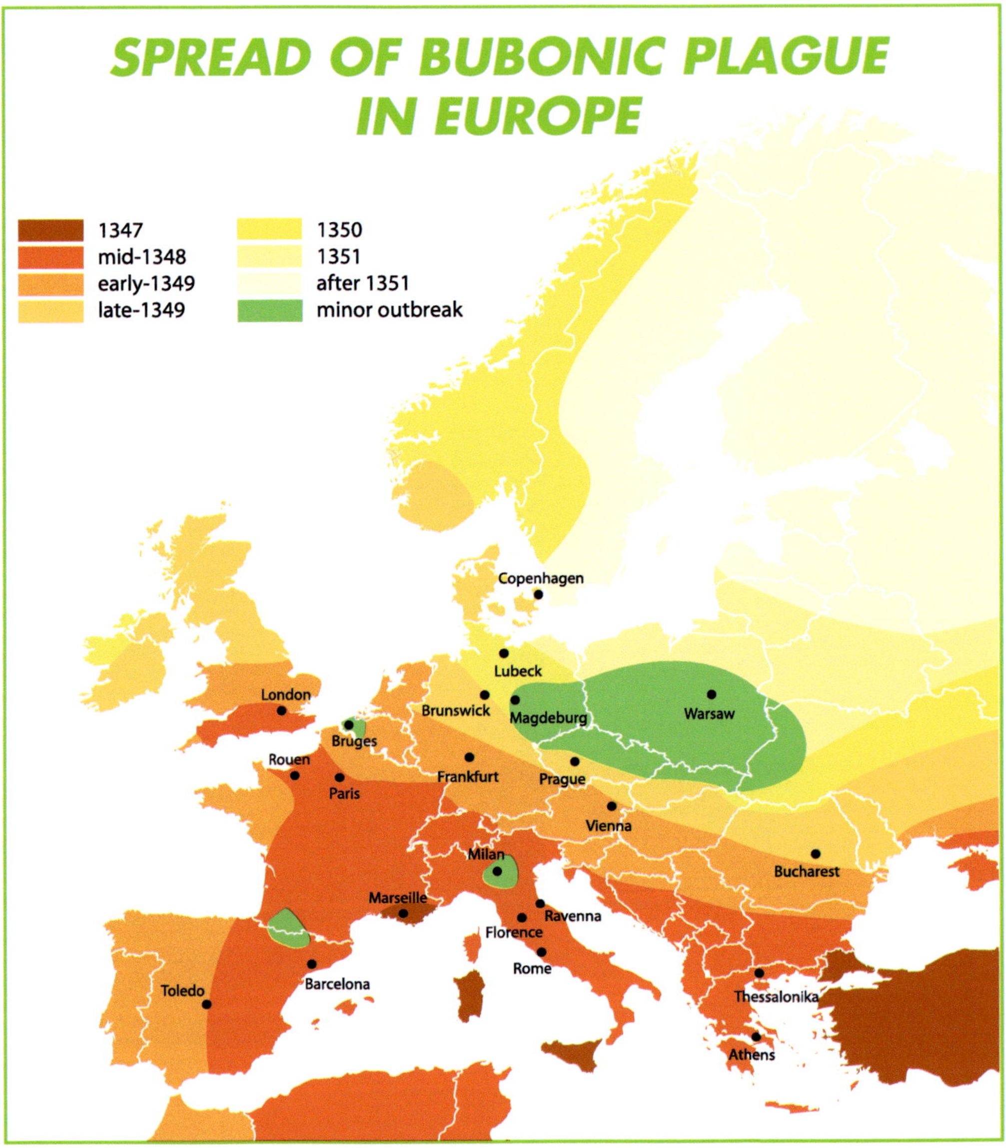

This map shows when and how plague likely spread across Europe according to some researchers.

HISTORY HAPPENED HERE: EAST SMITHFIELD CEMETERY OF LONDON

The East Smithfield cemetery in London, England, was excavated in the 1980s and discovered to contain bodies that date back to the time when the Black Death had ravaged London. Both mass graves and individual plots were uncovered. More than 500 bodies have been examined, and many more lay untouched.

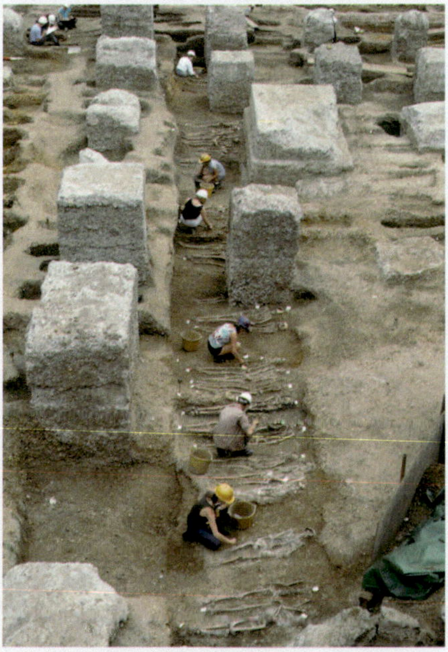

At East Smithfield cemetery, archaeologists worked carefully to uncover bodies of victims of the Black Death, more than 600 years after they were buried.

When the Black Death hit London, there were not enough cemeteries in the city to contain all of the dead. The land that became East Smithfield was purchased to contain the overflow of bodies, and there were *many* bodies. An estimated 30 to 50 percent of all people in London at the time died from plague. At the most deadly point of the Black Death there, 200 people were buried a day. That is why, in some of the mass graves at East Smithfield, the dead were buried in layers five bodies deep. The faster rate of deaths necessitated larger, more crowded graves.

Moscow was devastated between 1352 and 1353. The Russians recorded the same symptoms and high numbers of deaths as were experienced in the western European plague. The leader of eastern Russia, Grand Prince Ivanovich, died of plague and so did many members of his royal family.

Animal Victims

The Black Death did not just have a deadly impact on humankind. It also affected animals, both directly and indirectly. With farmers and farmhands dying, the livestock that they oversaw—including sheep, pigs, goats, chickens, and oxen—ran wild. Some animals contracted plague too.

English chronicler and eyewitness Henry Knighton wrote about the plight of the animals:

> *There was a great murrain [mass death] of sheep everywhere in the kingdom, so that in one place more than 5,000 sheep died in a single pasture; and they rotted so much that neither bird nor beast would approach them … Sheep and oxen strayed through the fields and among the crops, and there was none to drive them off or collect them, but they perished in uncounted numbers throughout all districts for lack of shepherds.*[6]

Wild animals, too, were caught in the pandemic. Large numbers caught the disease and passed it on throughout the natural world. With the disappearance of people, both dead and hiding from the disease, some animals ventured into areas they would normally avoid because of fear of people. One observer described being troubled by the aggressive behavior of wolves roaming around towns and villages in packs, hungrily searching for victims.

It seemed to all affected that the natural world was turned upside down. A man in Siena, Italy, who lost all five of his children to the Black Death, summed up what so many others thought about the horrific disaster. "No bells tolled [for the dead]," he wrote. "And nobody wept no matter what his loss because almost everyone expected death." Death had become an everyday occurrence for everyone. The man added, "People said and believed, 'This is the end of the world.'"[7]

How You See History

1. Why do people think the origins of the Black Death are still important?
2. Why do you think people started behaving differently as plague spread around them?
3. What other animals might have been affected by the Black Death? Explain how.

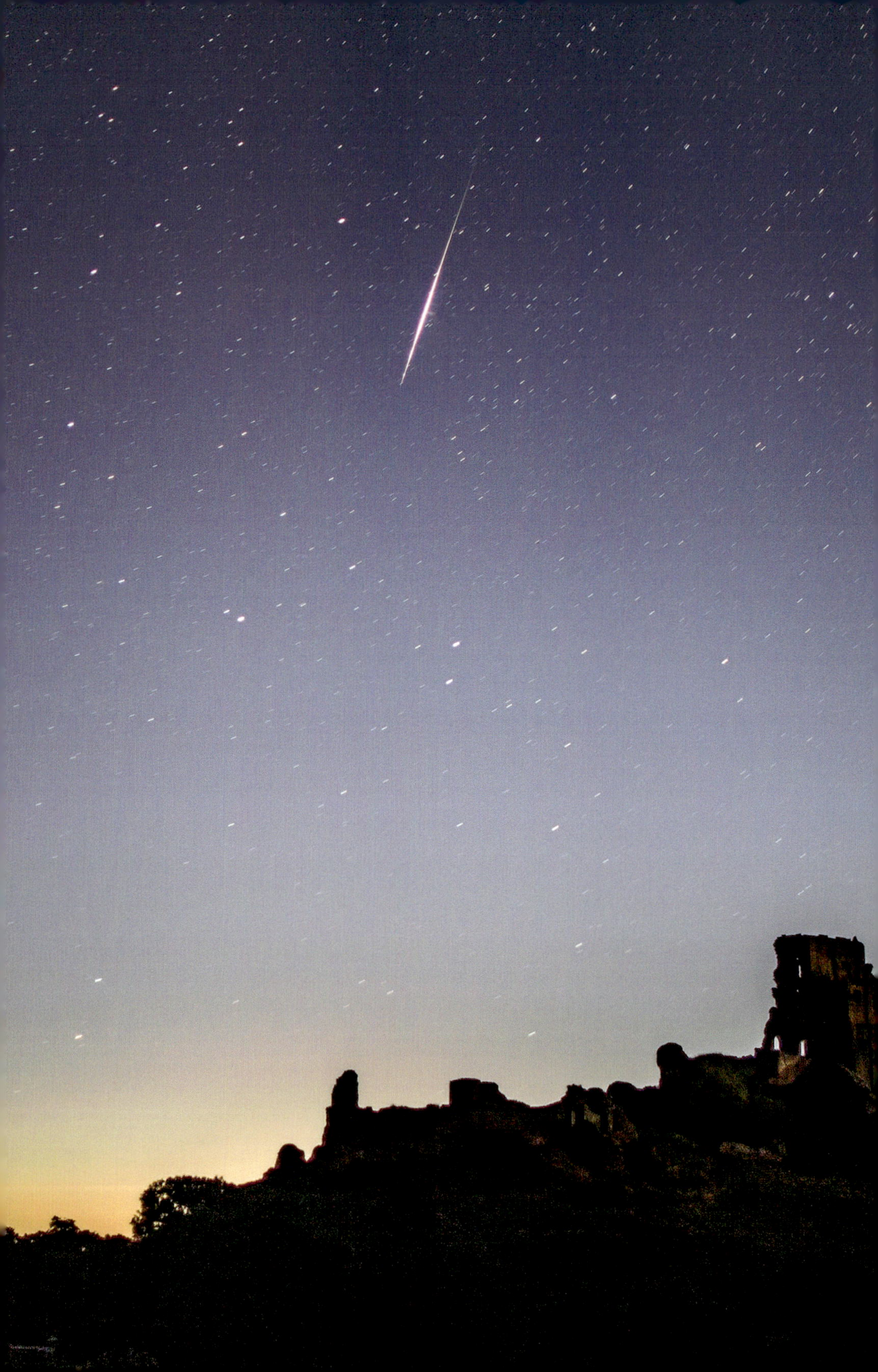

CHAPTER TWO

THE PUBLIC PANICS

Undoubtedly, the Black Death wreaked havoc in every place it traveled, including China, India, the Middle East, and farther. Much of the scholarship surrounding the pandemic focuses on Europe, which is how we know the various ways people of that time and region responded to the Black Death.

Some looked to astronomy, wondering if omens in the night skies had warned of an impending disaster. Many looked to religion for answers. Still others, finding no answers in their religion, turned away from their faith. A few tried to obtain solutions through science. However, since the medieval world knew little of modern science, their explanations and remedies were fruitless—and sometimes fatal. Some people became increasingly irrational and violent toward themselves or others, leading to the murders of thousands of innocent people.

Searching for Answers

In ancient and medieval times, it was common to look for omens that had preceded natural disasters, the birth of nobility, or other major events. As a terrible natural disaster, the spread of the Black Death motivated people to look for any signs that had come

A bright meteor in the sky was unusual enough that some people in medieval times thought it was an omen. When the Black Death appeared, they believed such an occurrence was a sign of bad events ahead.

before the pandemic. Some recalled that strangely heavy mists had blanketed several European regions in 1347. Others remembered seeing falling stars (which are nothing more than tiny meteors burning up in the atmosphere). A French friar named Jean de Venette described seeing a strange starlike object above Paris that broke into many pieces. Modern scholars think that de Venette and others witnessed a large meteor that broke into pieces as it raced through the atmosphere.

People were not only looking at shooting stars to explain the arrival of plague. For instance, some suggested that earthquakes had supposedly unleashed foul vapors from deep within the earth, which made humans sick when they inhaled them.

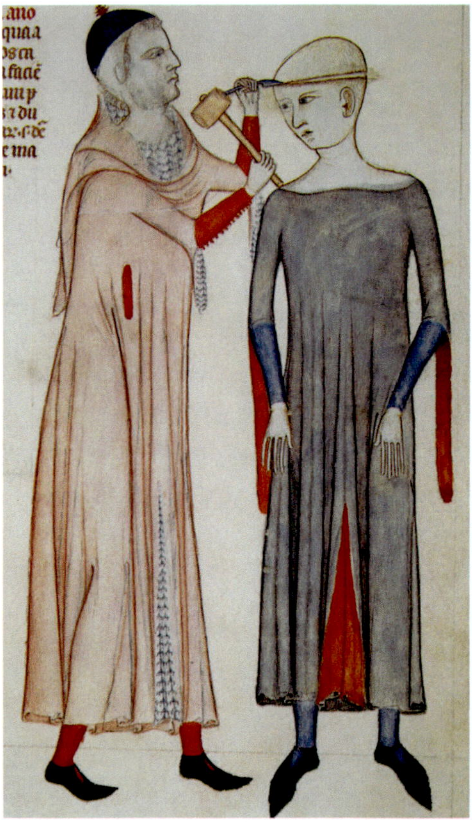

Medicine was not an exact science in the 14th century. Sometimes doctors made holes in people's heads, a practice called trepanation, to let out bad spirits or cure illnesses.

A number of people also blamed unnatural movements of the planets. They argued that this strange motion had caused the air on Earth to become corrupt and thereby infect humans with terrible sicknesses. This impure air hypothesis was supported by many intelligent scholars of the day, including noted physicians. In October 1348, a group of French doctors wrote:

> *Illnesses can be caused by the corruption of water or food … yet we still regard illnesses proceeding from the corruption of the air as much more dangerous. This is because bad air is more noxious [poisonous]*

than food or drink in that it can penetrate quickly to the heart and lungs to do its damage. We believe that the present epidemic or plague has arisen from air corrupt in its substance, and not changed in its attributes. By which we wish it [to] be understood that air, being pure and clear by nature, can only become putrid or corrupt by being mixed with something else, that is to say, with evil vapours.[1]

Many specialized doctors during this time truly believed that these "evil vapours" were the cause of the Black Death.

Sent by the Supernatural

Many reasons were given for the spread of plague, but none was more widespread than the idea that it was a punishment sent by God to force people to mend their wicked ways. However, God was not the only supernatural being blamed for bringing on plague. Respected scholar of medieval times Barbara W. Tuchman wrote:

Scandinavians believed that a Pest Maiden emerged from the mouth of the dead in the form of a blue flame and flew through the air to infect the next house. In Lithuania the Maiden was said to wave a red scarf through the door or window to let in the pest. One brave man, according to legend, deliberately waited at his open window with drawn sword and, at the fluttering of the scarf, chopped off the hand.

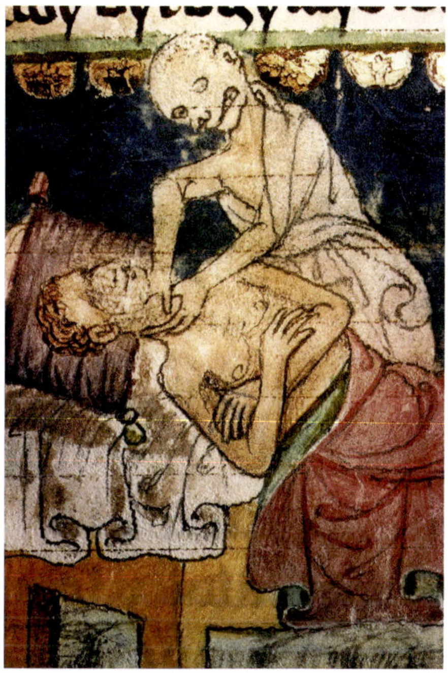

Without knowledge of modern medicine and how germs spread, people concocted explanations for why plague was spreading that made sense to them. In this image, a figure representing death attacks a plague victim.

He died of his deed, but his village was spared and the scarf [was] long preserved as a relic in the local church.[2]

These explanations, which seem so strange today, demonstrate the fact that medieval doctors had no clue as to what caused the epidemic.

Quarantines and Restrictions

Medieval doctors did not know how to give any sort of effective treatment to people who had the Black Death. On the other hand, it did seem apparent to doctors, as well as many ordinary people, that plague was somehow contagious. For this reason, a number of towns restricted travel and created rules for public hygiene and quarantines (the separation of plague victims from healthy people). While these new policies were not enough to stop the spread of the Black Death, they undoubtedly helped save some lives.

The Italian town of Pistoia issued anti-plague laws in May 1348. Among them was a decree that no citizen could go to the nearby cities of Pisa or Lucca. Similarly, no one was allowed to travel from those cities to Pistoia; if they did, they had to pay a hefty fine. Pistoia's rulers also passed laws that regulated the sale of meats and clothing to restrict and monitor goods coming in.

Authorities in Venice issued similar rules in 1348. Officials were selected to help maintain public health and hygiene efforts. Additionally, any foreign vessels were required to wait for 40 days before they could enter the Venetian harbor. (City officials could not predict how long the epidemic would last. This specific time period was chosen because it is the amount of time the Bible says that Jesus suffered in the wilderness.) Anyone who was sick or was showing symptoms inside the city was taken out to one of Venice's uninhabited islands to be quarantined.

Despite these earnest efforts, plague killed 100,000 people in Venice, which was roughly 60 percent of its residents. Among the dead were many doctors. Of those physicians who lived, most fled the city and left their patients to suffer in agony.

FROM THE SOURCE: PISTOIA'S RULES AND REGULATIONS

The Italian city of Pistoia was governed by a city council during the time of the Black Death. This group created many plague laws, some that seem strange today, including these:

> *VIII. Item. They have provided and ordered that in order to avoid useless or fruitless expenses no person should dare or presume to dress in new clothing during the period of mourning for any dead person or during the eight days after that …*
>
> *X. Item. So that the sounds of bells might not depress the infirm nor fear arise in them [the council] have provided and ordered that the bellringers or custodians in charge of the belltower of the cathedral of Pistoia shall not permit any bell … to be rung for the funeral of the dead nor shall any person dare or presume to ring any of these bells on the said occasion …*
>
> *XII. Item. They have provided and ordered that no person should dare … to raise or cause to be raised any wailing or clamor [loud crying] over any person or because of any person who has died outside the city, district or county of Pistoia; nor on the said occasion should any persons be brought together in any place except blood relatives and associates of such a dead person.*[1]

1. Quoted in "Pistoia," Fordham University Center for Medieval Studies, modified October 28, 1994, sourcebooks.fordham.edu/med/pistoia.asp.

All across Europe, similar attempts to stop the spread of plague emerged. These were all largely useless because there was no known cure, and no one realized that the disease was transmitted by fleas and rats. As a result, these disease carriers still came into contact with people and spread plague.

Unfounded Accusations

Because nothing substantial was known about the causes of the Black Death, many frightened and desperate people searched for someone to take the blame. These scapegoats were almost always viewed as abnormal and lived outside of mainstream society. Poor people and outsiders were targeted at times. Mentally ill and physically impaired people were also frequently suspected. According to scholar James C. Giblin:

> *On the edges of many villages, in poor huts made of sticks and straw, lived outcasts of various kinds. Some were deformed from birth, others were simple-minded, still others were insane. The villagers gave them names like Poor Tom and Mad Mag. The majority were harmless, although children sometimes taunted them and called the old women witches. Most adults simply left them alone. That changed when the Black Death came. As more people sickened and died, the survivors became increasingly frustrated. Neither the village priest nor the barber-surgeon had a solution for the plague … Maybe the children were right, the fearful survivors thought. Maybe Mad Mag really was a witch. If they got rid of her, maybe the pestilence would finally go away.*[3]

The biggest group that medieval Europeans blamed for the Black Death was the Jewish people. They were accused of many things during this time period, including poisoning wells and other supplies of drinking water in order to exterminate Christians. More than 200 Jewish communities were destroyed, and thousands of people were killed.

Unjust Persecution

It is only natural to wonder why so many people believed Jews had caused the terrible pandemic. Based on traditional Christian teachings and the Bible, Jews were responsible for the death of Jesus Christ. As a result, most Europeans, being devoted Christians, were willing to believe almost anything bad about their Jewish neighbors, even the false ideas that Jews drank the blood of Christian children.

THEY MADE HISTORY: POPE CLEMENT VI

Pope Clement VI was born Pierre Roger in 1291 in France. Beginning his religious life as a monk, he rose in the ranks of the Catholic Church until he became pope in 1342. He watched over the Church from the city of Avignon. He was responsible for a crusade (a religious war) in 1344 to capture land in the Middle East from Muslims.

As pope, Clement rejected his previous vow of poverty and lived in a palace with great wealth. When the Black Death struck his city, it entered the pope's home as well. Perhaps about one-fourth of his staff died. Meanwhile, Clement's doctors instructed him to sit between two large fires at all times. Although the doctors did not know how plague spread, making the pope do this may have kept the fleas away since the insects would have avoided such extreme heat.

Still, Clement was active during the Black Death in his own way. He worked to make sure that people had places to be buried. He assured his followers that all who died could go to heaven. He also issued two decrees that Jewish people should not be blamed for plague or punished. He presented rational explanations why, though many Christians refused to listen. Clement VI died in 1352 of an illness unrelated to plague.

The reigning pope, Clement VI, tried to use simple logic to explain why Jews could not be guilty of causing plague. He first pointed out that large numbers of Jews were dying of the disease. Why, he asked, would they want to kill so many of their own kind? Moreover, numerous regions where no Jews lived were also struck by plague, so there had to be some other cause. In an attempt to reduce violence, Pope Clement declared that no Christian should try to hurt or kill Jews. Unfortunately, anti-Semitism (prejudice against Jews) was so powerful in Europe that very few people listened to or obeyed the pope. Huge numbers of innocent Jews were massacred by angry mobs between 1348 and 1350.

Sometimes Jews confessed to poisoning wells after being tortured. However, obviously untrue admissions such as these gave townspeople across Europe another excuse to continue to persecute and kill Jewish people. The following account from the German town of Strasbourg told how local Jews were burned alive in February 1349:

> *They burnt the Jews on a wooden platform in their cemetery. There were about two thousand of them. Those who wanted*

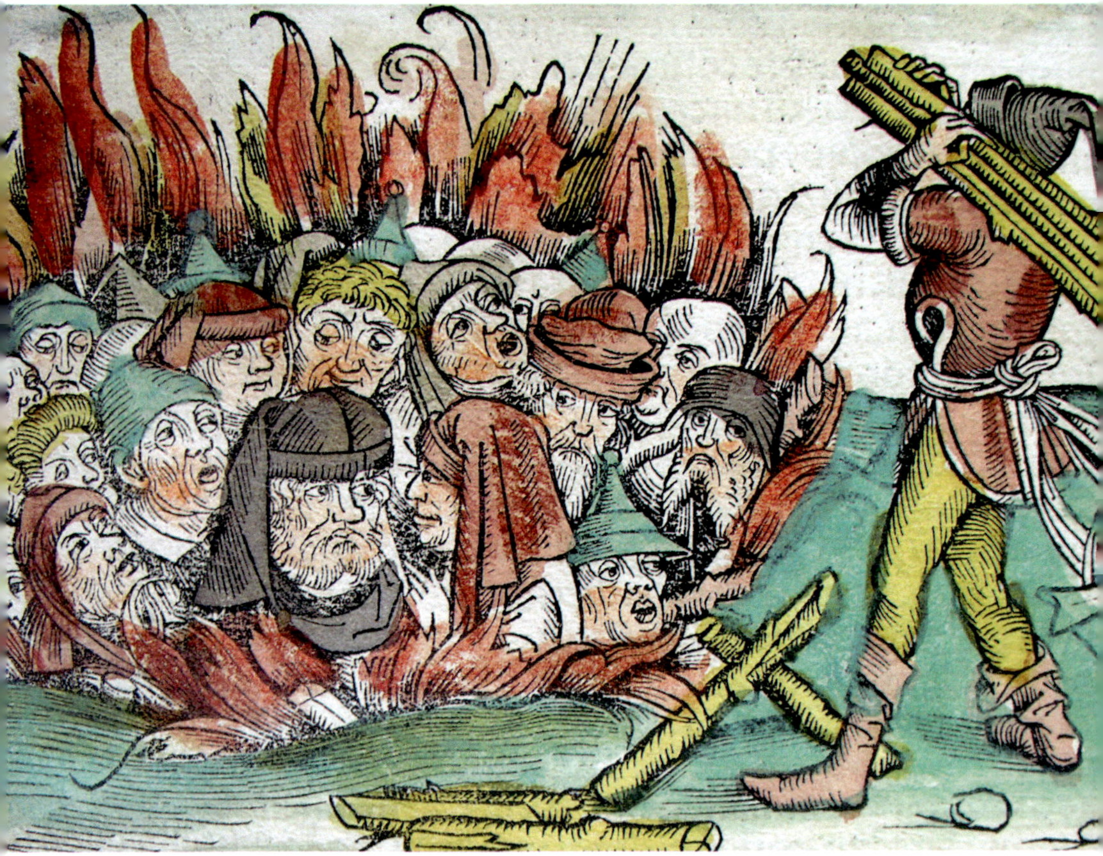

Jewish people were terribly and unfairly persecuted in the 1300s—and beyond. Shown here is an image depicting Jewish people being burned alive in a town in present-day Germany.

PAST MEETS PRESENT: ANTI-SEMITISM

Anti-Semitism did not arise during the Black Death, nor, unfortunately, did it end when the plague died out. Jewish people have long been the object of prejudice. The origin of anti-Semitism lies in the differences between the Jewish religion and other religions. When the Christian Church became powerful in many places, the Jewish people suffered. Unfair laws often kept them from becoming accepted members of communities. In medieval times, Jews were not given many of the rights that others had. Sometimes, they had to live in separate parts of cities. Still, many managed to rise in society—through trade, banking, and other businesses. Success brought jealousy and more prejudice at times. In some places, Jews were forced to leave their countries.

In later history, even as laws began to call for an end to anti-Semitic practices and religious organizations like the Catholic Church denounced anti-Semitism, it continued in many places. Jews were violently attacked in Russia in planned campaigns called pogroms in the late 1800s and early 1900s. The Jewish people suffered through the Holocaust during World War II (1939–1945), when Nazi Germany sought to eliminate them. In modern times, anti-Semitism is often not as blatant, but the Jewish people—those who practice the Jewish religion and ethnic Jews—continue to face it and fight against it.

to baptize themselves [as Christians] were spared. Many small children were taken out of the fire and baptized against the will of their fathers and mothers. And everything that was owed to the Jews was cancelled … The [town] council, however, took the cash that the Jews possessed and divided it among the working-men proportionately … After this wealth was divided among the artisans some gave their share to the Cathedral or to the Church on the advice of their confessors ... In some towns they burnt the Jews after a trial, in others, without a trial. In some cities the Jews themselves set fire to their houses.[4]

Modern scholars note this time period for being especially dark for European Jews. Despite being killed by the same disease as everyone else, their neighbors turned on them and blamed them for the Black Death.

The Flagellants

When none of their actions were able to stop the pandemic, some people appealed directly to God. However, when the plague deaths continued, they soon came to feel that their prayers were being ignored.

Some of the most devout Christians joined groups of flagellants, a name that comes from the word "flagellate," which means to punish by whipping. Groups of several hundred flagellants traveled from town to town and put on a kind of show. They would head directly to the local church or city center and beat themselves with a special whip with iron spikes that was called a scourge. According to an eyewitness, Henry of Herford, a scourge was "a kind of stick from which three tails with large knots hung down. Through the knots were thrust iron spikes ... With such scourges they lashed themselves on their ... bodies so that they became swollen and blue."[5] These beatings were supposed to re-create the whippings Jesus received before his crucifixion. Flagellants believed that their suffering would convince God to be merciful and stop the spread of the Black Death.

However, this first session of whipping was only the beginning of a typical flagellant ceremony. Next, the worshippers sang dirges (sad songs). Following this, it was common for the flagellants to lie down on the ground. Two of them then walked back and forth among the ones on the ground, beating them with scourges. Then, the men on the ground stood up and began beating themselves again. The final step of their demonstration was to listen as one of the masters gave what was known as the Flagellants' Sermon. The flagellants claimed that these sermons were the words of an angel sent by God. They warned that everyone in Europe was a sinner and the only way to stop the Black Death was to follow God's ways.

At first, many of the townsfolk who watched this strange public display admired the dedication of the flagellants. They donated money or allowed the flagellants to stay in their homes. The most extreme believers even joined the movement and traveled across the countryside. Over time, however, people grew tired of the self-torturers. Because the flagellants claimed that their

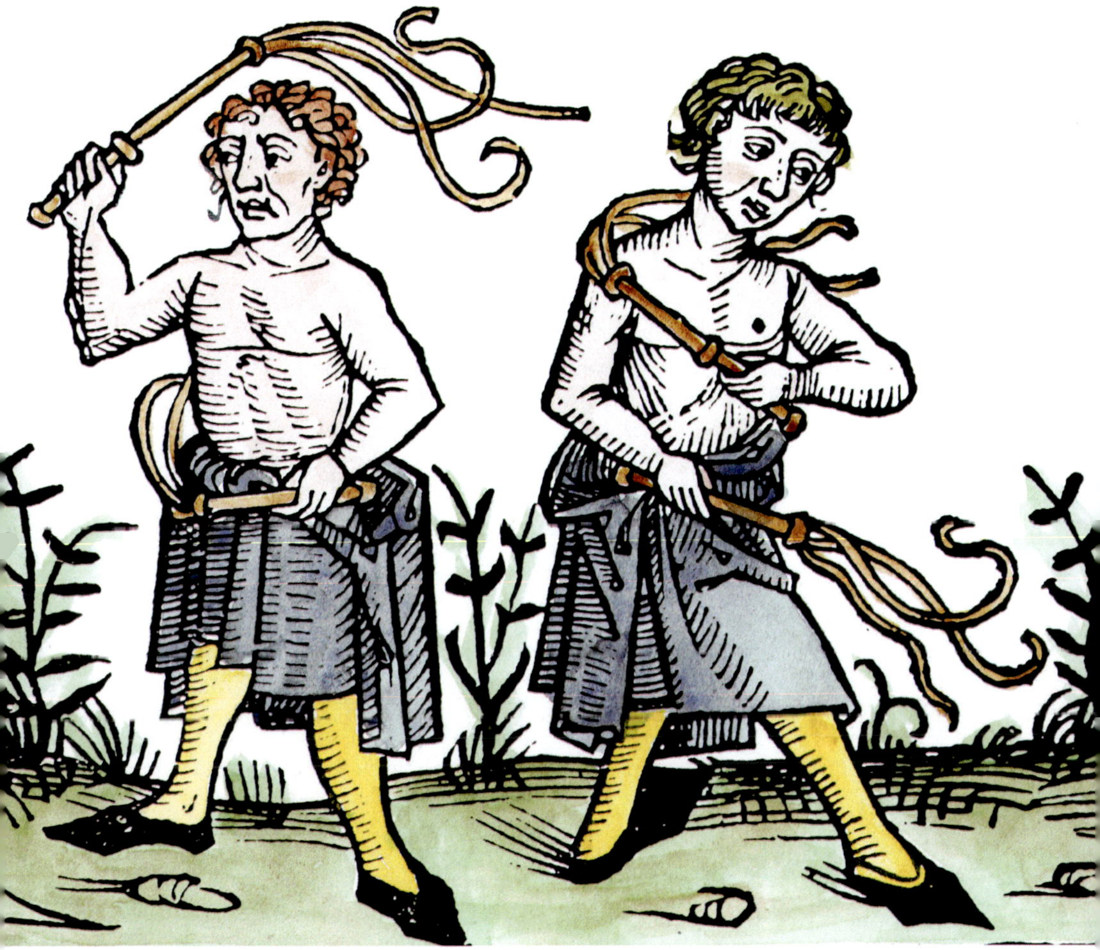

Flagellants believed they were making up for their sins by whipping themselves. This practice has not completely died out.

sacrifices would prevent plague, it looked bad when large numbers of them caught the disease and died. They were shown to be just as vulnerable to the Black Death as anyone else.

Moreover, the flagellants had become a threat to the central Catholic Church. In October 1349, Pope Clement VI issued a statement that said the flagellants were not supported by God or the Church. Influential local churchmen also made similar speeches. Town mayors and councils began denying the groups entrance to their cities. As a result of these efforts, the wandering groups steadily disbanded.

Unstoppable

Unsurprisingly, the actions of flagellants and others trying to fight the Black Death without scientific reasoning failed miserably. The incredibly large numbers of deaths continued into the early 1350s. Otto Friedrich, a leading expert on plague, summed up Europe's wreckage:

> *The chronicles of the fourteenth century [present] an image of deserted cottages falling in ruins and untilled wheat fields reverting to wilderness. Thousands of villages all across the face of Europe did simply disappear. The buried remnants are faintly visible in aerial photographs, spectral outlines of a vanished people.*[6]

Some areas of Europe saw population losses of 80 percent, while others were barely touched by fatalities. French writer Jean Froissart estimated that 33 percent of the continent's inhabitants were wiped out, or about 25 million people. For comparison, one of the deadliest pandemics in modern history—the Spanish flu of the early 1900s—killed about 3 percent of the world's population. Archaeological evidence supports the Black Death's startling percentages, though.

Those who did not die of the Black Death had many questions about what had happened and whether it would happen again. One of their most urgent questions—what was the cause?—was not answered until hundreds of years later.

HISTORY HAPPENED HERE: COSMESTON MEDIEVAL VILLAGE

Cosmeston Medieval Village is located in the country of Wales in the United Kingdom. It is a re-creation of a community that was abandoned around the time of the Black Death. Even if it was not plague that killed people in the village, they may have had to leave Cosmeston to find work in larger towns and cities soon after. It is an example of how communities changed because of the Black Death.

Cosmeston's ruins became buried and overgrown over the years. In fact, no one knew a village was there for hundreds of years. An archaeological dig around a nearby lake in the 1980s led to its discovery. Local people decided the unearthing was an opportunity to teach others about life in medieval times. Today, rebuilt stone houses and actors dressed as medieval villagers give visitors an understanding of what life was like in Wales in the middle part of the 14th century.

How You See History

1. Why do you think Venice's quarantine efforts failed to stop the spread of plague?
2. Why do you think some Christians disobeyed the pope's order not to persecute the Jewish people?
3. Why do you think the flagellants attracted and then lost their following?

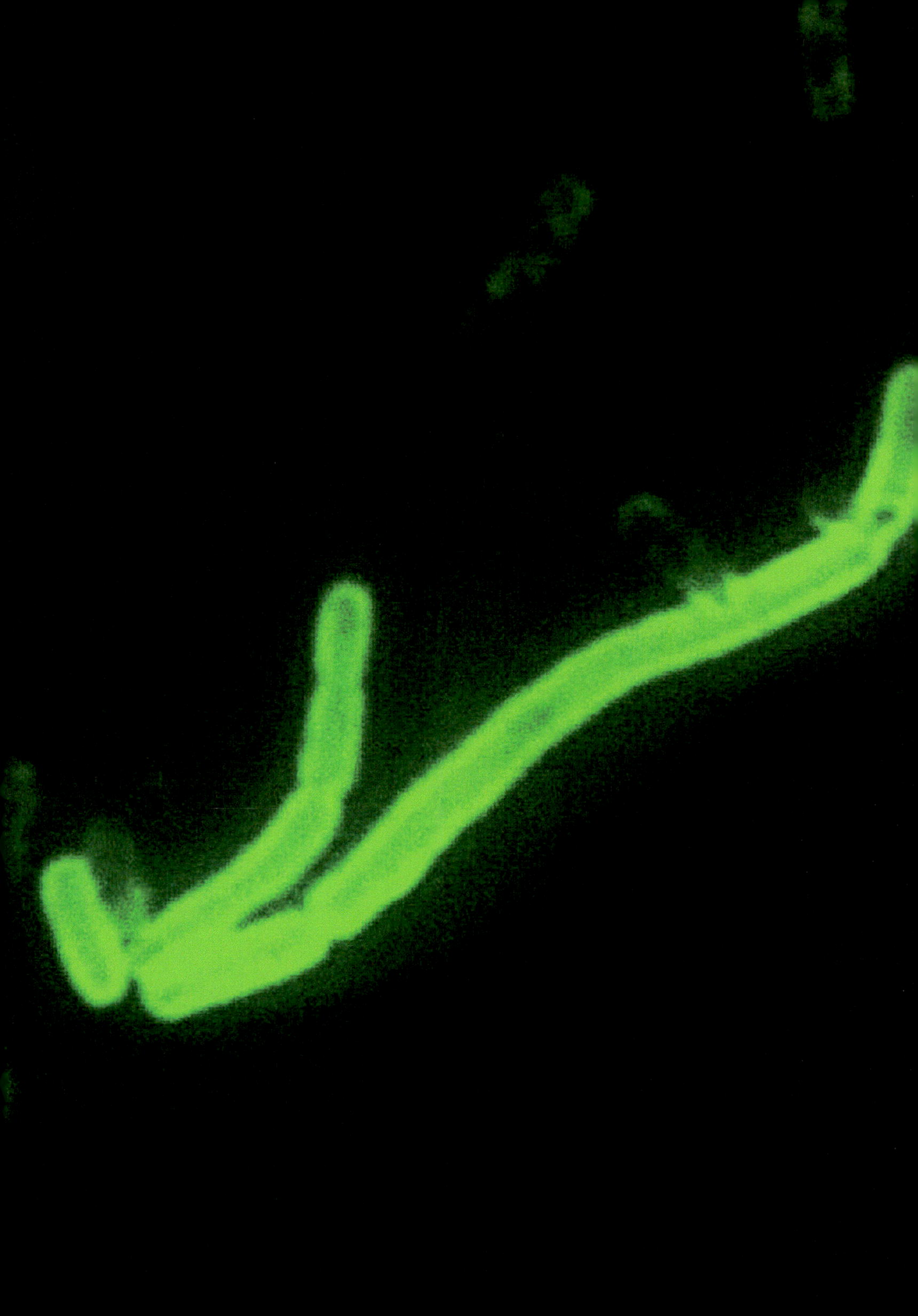

CHAPTER THREE

FINDING THE CAUSE

Students of world history are struck by the Black Death's lethalness, its wildfire-like spread, and its ramifications on society. They may not be as familiar with the cause of the Black Death. Nearly all medieval doctors were completely in the dark about the source of the disease. Subsequently, these doctors' methods of containing the outbreak and treating the disease were woefully inadequate—sometimes causing patients to die before plague could kill them.

Scientific advances beginning in the 17th and 18th centuries led scientists to learn more about the invisible world of microbes, laying the groundwork for other scientists to introduce the germ theory in the 1800s. This idea hypothesized that germs could invade the human body and cause disease. Today, that seems obvious. However, at that time, many scientists would not believe such a concept. After experiments proved the groundbreaking theory, researchers began discerning which germs caused which diseases, including the one that caused the Black Death.

Most medical researchers and historians agree that the cause of the Black Death was *Yersinia pestis*. In his book *The*

Today, we know the Black Death's cause. This is a view of the plague bacterium *Yersinia pestis*, as seen under a microscope.

Black Death and the Transformation of the West, scholar David Herlihy provided an explanation of the research of the 1890s:

> *In 1894, in China, the plague emerged from the inland provinces of Hunan and Canton, where it was endemic [widespread], to attack the port city of Hong Kong ... A Swiss microbiologist named Alexandre Yersin ... hurried to Hong Kong and set up a laboratory there, in hopes of containing the disease before it struck southeast Asia. In 1894 he isolated the bacillus [plague germ] and went on to develop a serum for the treatment of plague. The disease is consequently called ...* Yersinia pestis, *after Alexandre Yersin.*[1]

Research about the bubonic plague did not stop with Yersin's discovery. Other scientists worked on answering questions about how plague germs are passed along and why the disease seemingly disappeared and then reappeared years later. Even today, scientists study *Yersinia pestis* in search of new discoveries to fill the holes in the history of the Black Death. There are many facts that have already been established, however.

Always Around

One of the first things researchers noticed about bubonic plague, or the bacterium *Yersinia pestis*, is that it naturally affects rats and other rodents—not humans. Outbreaks in human populations, experts say, are much less common than those in animal populations. Scientists have found that at any given time, a few rodents or other small creatures in a handful of remote wilderness areas are carrying the disease. These small groups of animals make up what medical experts call a disease reservoir. Most of the time, the animals in disease reservoirs have too few bacteria in their systems to kill them or to cause the illness to spread. In other words, plague sleeps in these carriers. For a few years, decades, or in some cases centuries, it remains trapped and dormant in its reservoir, as if waiting for the perfect moment to escape.

Evidence shows that, on occasion, plague germs living in one or more wild animals become numerous enough to begin spreading from one animal to another. Most often, this happens by way of fleas that live in animals' fur.

FROM THE SOURCE: AN EARLY FORM OF GERM THEORY

Contrary to popular opinion, not all medieval doctors were totally unaware of what causes most diseases. Two brilliant 14th-century Islamic scholars, Ibn Khatima and Ibn al-Khatib, proposed an early theory of what they called "infection." Although not precisely the germ theory introduced in the 19th century by European scientists, this early version was partially correct and far ahead of its time:

> *To those who say, "How can we admit the possibility of infection while the religious law denies it?" we reply that the existence of contagion is established by experience, investigation, the evidence of the senses and trustworthy reports. These facts constitute a sound argument. The fact of infection becomes clear to the investigator who notices how he who establishes contact with the afflicted [sick person] gets the disease, whereas he who is not in contact remains safe, and how transmission is effected through garments, vessels and earrings.*[1]

1. Quoted in Philip K. Hitti, *History of the Arabs* (London, UK: Macmillan, 1970), p. 576.

A common kind of flea is *Xenopsylla cheopis*, which is also called the Oriental rat flea. This flea consumes its host's blood, which may contain plague bacteria. The germs have little or no effect on fleas, but they manage to spread when a carrier flea lands on and bites an uninfected animal. The process rapidly repeats itself, and the result can be an epidemic among wild creatures.

When these infected animals remain isolated from human civilization, the disease will run its course and eventually begin to subside. However, when the infected animals come into contact with humans, a very different scenario takes place. As scholar James C. Giblin explained, this is how bubonic plague in the 1300s most likely spread from rodents in remote sections of central Asia to people:

Although it was only an eighth of an inch long, the rat flea was a tough, adaptable creature. It depended for nourishment on the blood of its host, which it obtained through a daggerlike snout that could pierce the rat's skin. And in its stomach the flea often carried thousands of the deadly bacteria that caused the bubonic plague … A black rat could tolerate a moderate amount of them [germs], too, without showing ill effects. But sometimes the flea contained so many bacteria that they invaded the rat's lungs or nervous system when the flea injected its snout. Then the rat died a swift and horrible death, and the flea had to find a new host.

Aiding the tiny flea in its search were its powerful legs, which could jump more than 150 times the creature's length. In most instances the flea landed on another black rat … If most of the rats in the vicinity were already dead or dying from the plague, the flea might leap to a human being instead.[2]

Symptoms of Infection

After making the fateful jump to a person, the hungry flea immediately bit its new host in search of blood. In the 1300s, this was probably a hunter or a trader who perhaps felt a slight pinch. They did not realize that this innocent bite signaled the initial attack of an invisible but deadly invasion force. During the feeding process, the insect transferred some plague germs into the bite wound. The bacteria worked their way into the person's lymph nodes. (These organs contain cells that help the body's immune system fight foreign invaders, including germs.) The *Yersinia pestis* germs found the lymph nodes to be ideal places to multiply. Soon, they created colonies that increased in size, and within three to eight days, the germs formed lumps the size of eggs or larger. These lumps were the buboes that numerous medieval writers mentioned when describing the classic symptoms of the Black Death. Most often, the buboes appeared in the underarms or the groin.

After several more days had passed, the germs reached the victim's bloodstream. The bloodstream transported the germs to the vital organs, including the lungs. Soon, dark spots appeared on the skin, and in many cases, blood oozed from the skin as well. Next,

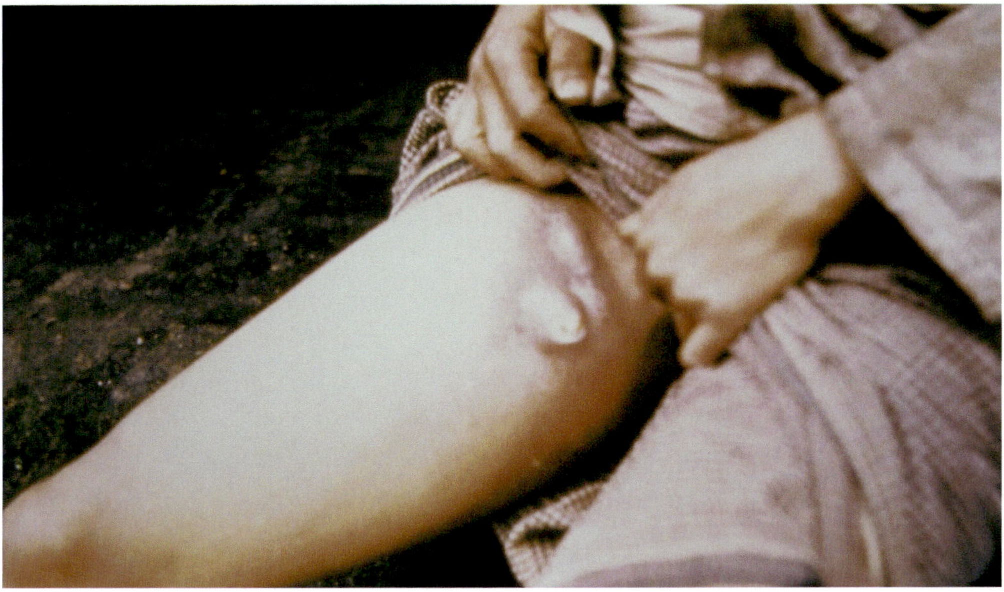

The raised lumps on plague victims' bodies, called buboes, are a sign of infection.

Giblin wrote, "the nervous system started to collapse, causing dreadful pain [in the limbs] and bizarre movements of the arms and legs. Then, as death neared, the mouth gaped open and the skin blackened from internal bleeding."[3]

The death of the victim was not the end of the process, however. The next phase in the lethal cycle began after death. Just as the infected fleas had earlier jumped off their dead rat hosts, the fleas now left behind the dead human ones. Still full of *Yersinia pestis*, the fleas searched for, and sometimes found, a new human host. From hunters and traders to sailors, city dwellers, farmers, and others, the germs ravaged one host after another.

Most modern experts agree that the Black Death followed this general scenario. The main evidence used to support this view is that the medieval writers described symptoms identical or at least very similar to those seen in modern cases of plague.

Examining the Evidence

Medieval descriptions of the Black Death have long been interesting to epidemiologists, scientists who study disease origins and transmission. Epidemiologists track down and study clues to the various ways that germs spread disease. For them, it was not enough to know how the plague bacteria made it out of an animal reservoir in central Asia and infected humans. It is obvious that those infected people proceeded to carry the deadly germs to one or more nearby towns. Epidemiologists wanted to know much more. They wanted to be able to trace, as best as they could, the course of the Black Death as it made its way through the Middle East and Europe. Piecing together this chain of evidence would help modern scientists better understand this killer disease and thereby keep it from causing a new wave of Black Death.

Fortunately for medical researchers, historians had already started piecing together the important string of events that caused the spread of the Black Death. That chain began in Kaffa, the Crimean port city that was attacked by the Mongols early in 1346. The residents of Kaffa were naturally concerned when the enemy started lobbing diseased corpses over the city's walls. They were aware that these bodies were causing them to come down with a terrible sickness, but they had no idea how the disease was spreading among them. They had no clue that the disease they were experiencing followed unique paths of infection.

There were two key carriers that spread the Black Death beyond Kaffa: rats and people on whom one or more fleas had made a temporary home. Although it was the fleas that carried the actual plague germs, they could not have made it out of the city and onto ships without rats and humans to carry them.

Of these two carriers, the rats were by far the most numerous and ultimately lethal. Indeed, a major reason that the disease was able to spread so quickly from one city or country to another was that no one suspected that rats were carrying the disease. After all, they were practically everywhere. Rats and other rodents scrounged for food in farmers' fields and barns, grain supplies, houses, shops, ships, and elsewhere. People had accepted them as pesky but ever-present nuisances. They never suspected that the rats were helping the transmission of the Black Death from place to place.

No one took notice as rats, some carrying infected fleas, crawled from docks onto ships. The ships took these live disease-carriers from Kaffa to ports near and far. Harbormasters in a city that had not yet encountered the disease often ordered the crews and passengers of newly arrived ships to stay onboard. This is what happened when Genoese ships from the East reached the southern Italian port of

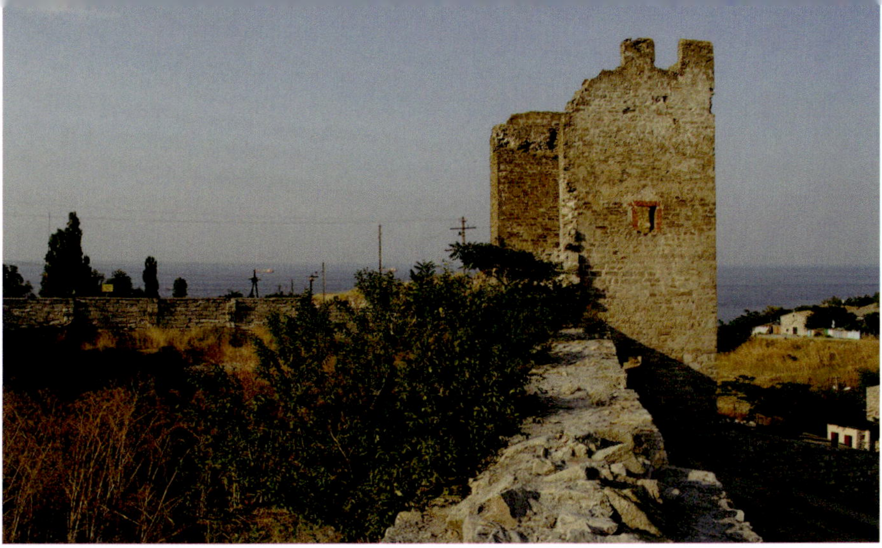

The medieval town of Kaffa is now called Feodosiya (or Feodosia). It is located in southern Ukraine.

Messina. However, the strategy of keeping potentially infected people from leaving the ships did not prevent the spread of plague. It is likely that infected rats got to land by running along the ropes that tied the ships to the docks.

Forms of the Disease

Once the rats carrying the infected fleas entered Messina and other port cities, the next step in plague's assault on Europe took place. Some fleas hopped off the rats and found human hosts. Many of those new hosts caught plague. When those victims died, the fleas jumped to either other humans or animals and spread the contagion in all directions.

For the people infected with plague, there were three possible forms for the disease to take. The most common was the passage of *Yersinia pestis* from the lymph nodes to the major organs of the body, producing the symptoms described previously. Medical experts generally refer to this form of the illness, which was fatal in 50 to 60 percent of cases, as bubonic plague.

In a minority of cases, however, the disease could take two other forms. The first is called pneumonic plague, because it involves a rare kind of pneumonia. Sometimes, when an infected person is exposed to a sudden and sharp drop in temperature, the germs can move into the lungs. The victim rapidly develops a severe cough

THEY MADE HISTORY: GUY DE CHAULIAC

Many medieval doctors died of the bubonic plague during the Black Death. The fact that they had no knowledge or ability to stop the epidemic was a tremendous embarrassment to those who managed to survive. Guy de Chauliac was a distinguished French physician of that time. Born around 1300, he was perhaps the most famous doctor in Europe, tending to Pope Clement VI as well as two other popes. He also wrote a widely read book about performing surgery that was used for nearly 300 years. The Frenchman was among the first people to describe two different types of plague, pneumonic and bubonic, helping historians today understand more about the outbreak. In one of his works, de Chauliac described plague from a doctor's point of view at the time:

> *The plague was shameful for the physicians, who could give no help at all, especially as, out of fear of infection, they hesitated to visit the sick. Even if they did, they achieved nothing.*[1]

Guy de Chauliac survived the Black Death, but died July 25, 1368, in Avignon, France.

1. Quoted in John Withington, *Disaster! A History of Earthquakes, Floods, Plagues, and Other Catastrophes* (New York, NY: Skyhorse Publishing, 2010), p. 115.

and begins spitting up bloody mucus. Because the mucus contains plague microbes, it can infect other people or animals directly when it flies into the air or lands on nearby objects. It is therefore extremely contagious and dangerous. Almost every case of pneumonic plague during the time of the Black Death was fatal.

The third and rarest form of the disease, septicemic plague, occurs when the bacteria enter the bloodstream immediately and in huge numbers. As the germs move through the body, they multiply quickly. Within hours, they infect all areas of the body, resulting in

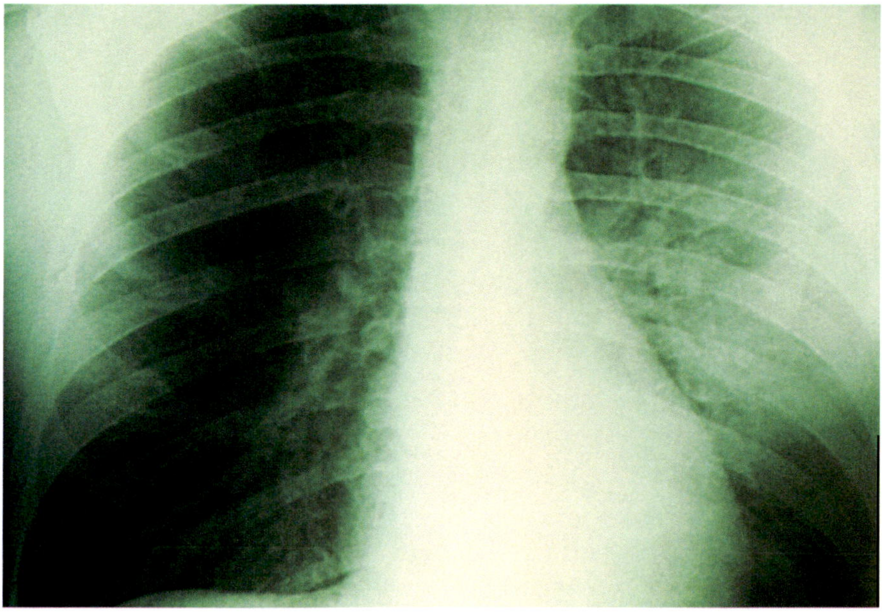

This X-ray of a patient with pneumonic plague reveals an infection in both lungs. Pneumonic plague is a form of plague that can be passed from person to person by breathing in airborne droplets.

death in less than one day. British scholar Philip Ziegler wrote about septicemic plague:

> *The victim is dead long before buboes have had time to form. It is in this form of plague that* Pulex irritans, *the man-borne flea, has a chance to operate. So rich in bacilli [plague germs] is the blood of a sick man that the flea can easily infect itself and carry on the disease to a new prey without the need of a rat to provide fresh sources of infection. Septicaemic [septicemic] plague must have been the rarest of the three interwoven diseases which composed the Black Death but it was certainly as lethal as its pneumonic cousin and it introduced yet another means by which the plague could settle itself in a new area and spread hungrily among the inhabitants.*[4]

Escaping Infection

It is important to note that some people in the 1300s, as well as in outbreaks of plague in later eras, were exposed to the disease but did not contract it. The Black Death seemed to kill randomly. Often, it wiped out entire families or neighborhoods and villages. In other instances, people did not contract plague despite being in close contact with the infected.

Experts point to a number of reasons for this. First, the most frequent form, bubonic plague, was rarely contagious from person to person. The main carrier was infected fleas, so a person's chances of getting sick depended on their exposure to the fleas, not the infected human. Therefore, the disease spread more easily in areas with poor sanitation, where more diseased fleas and rats were likely to gather. In areas where homes and streets were cleaner, more people escaped infection. Moreover, because the deadly fleas often inhabited animal fur, people who had minimal contact with animals were less likely to get sick.

An even more important factor affecting plague's ability to spread was personal immunity. Modern medical researchers have found that, for a variety of reasons, some people have stronger immune systems than others. Thus, a person with a strong immune system had a good chance of fighting off the infection, especially if their exposure was relatively light. As a result of these factors and others, some who were directly exposed to people suffering from the Black Death did not catch it.

Ineffective Treatments

If medieval doctors had known how germs work, or about fleas' role in transmission, lives could have been saved. However, the germ theory and research of later doctors and scientists were still hundreds of years in the future.

In the Middle Ages, many doctors based their treatments on those of an ancient Greek physician named Galen. He did studies in his own time to come up with theories about the human body, and many later doctors accepted his ideas without question and applied them as they wanted, with little scientific basis to back their actions. For example, Galen claimed illness could be related to someone's personality, eating or drinking to excess, and even the temperature of the air. Another supposed cause of illness was a miasma, which is a term for a pocket of air that is harmful or poisonous.

HISTORY HAPPENED HERE: ST. MARY'S ASHWELL

For those who are interested in learning about the Black Death through medieval graffiti, a British church has some well-preserved scrawls in Latin and Old English. St. Mary's Ashwell is a church in the village of Ashwell, Hertfordshire, north of London, England. It was first built in the 1300s and stands in good condition today. Over hundreds of years, priests, architects, and others who have spent time within the building inscribed messages on its stone walls and pillars. A translated piece of writing about the plague period reads:

There was a plague
1000, three times 100, five times 10,
a pitiable, fierce violent
(plague departed); a wretched populace survives to witness and in the end
a mighty wind, Maurus, thunders in this year in the world, 1361[1]

The writing tells us that the Black Death arrived in the village in "1000, three times 100, five times 10," which means the year 1350. Plague likely left briefly and then reoccurred, not completely disappearing from the community until 1361, as noted.

1. Quoted in "Decoding the Graffiti—The Large Letters," St. Mary's Ashwell, www.stmarysashwell.org.uk/church/graffiti/decode.htm (accessed May 11, 2020).

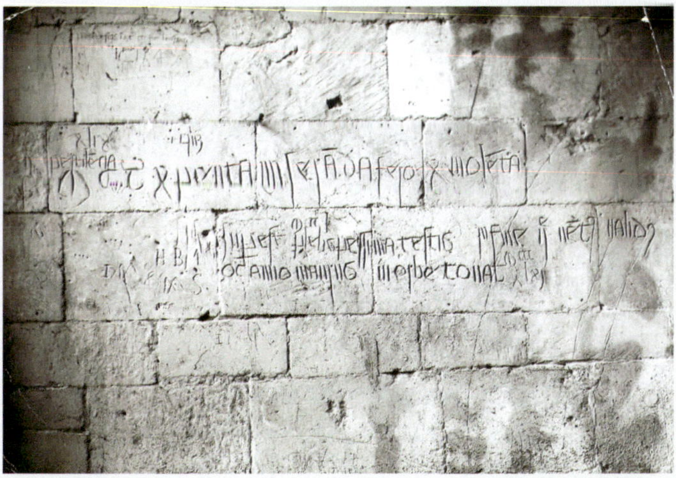

St. Mary's Ashwell is constructed of chalk stone, which made carving into its surfaces easy.

PAST MEETS PRESENT: EXAMINING THE PLAGUE OF THE PAST

Some people today do not accept that the Black Death was plague. They think other diseases are more likely responsible for the high numbers of fatalities and rapid spread. For example, the modern virus that causes Ebola is highly contagious from person to person, causes hemorrhaging (the loss of huge quantities of blood), and has a high fatality rate. Further, the modern strain of the *Yersinia pestis* bacterium, while dangerous when untreated, is unlikely to be as virulent as the Black Death seems to have been.

To solve this mystery, in 2011, scientists studied the remains of Black Death victims that were found in East Smithfield, one of the few cemeteries that is known for certain to contain plague victims. The scientists studied DNA found in the victims' teeth. While they confirmed the bacterium in the bodies was *Yersinia pestis,* its DNA was slightly different than the modern *Yersinia pestis* bacterium. That slight difference suggests that it is possible the *Yersinia pestis* bacterium of the Black Death was a more lethal and contagious mutation, which—luckily—seems to have disappeared.

Some medieval doctors believed an evil miasma was the cause of the Black Death, so they recommended hanging sweet-smelling flowers or herbs throughout homes. Other harmless—but ineffective—remedies included sleeping during the day rather than at night, avoiding southern winds, and simply not thinking about illness and disease.

For those already sick with plague, doctors tried some deadly treatments, such as bloodletting. This meant opening veins, especially those near buboes, and allowing "bad" blood to drain out of the body. Unsurprisingly, this only made the patient weaker and less able to fight the infection. Lancing and draining the buboes was also common. While this might have rid the body of some bacteria (unbeknownst to the doctors), bacteria remained and continued to multiply.

Many doctors applied various substances to the buboes in an effort to reduce them or draw out poison. One such mixture contained tree resin, lily roots, and human excrement. Other patients were told to drink crushed emeralds mixed with water. Still others were directed to ingest arsenic or mercury, toxins that were more likely to kill the patient than plague bacteria. There were many other useless "cures" during this time. Helpless, desperate patients would try anything.

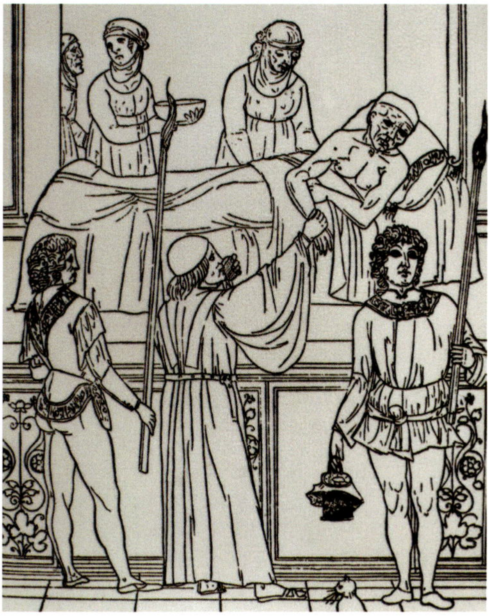

In this medieval engraving, a doctor treats a plague victim. The doctor holds a pomander, which is a container for fragrant plants, in front of his nose. Its scent was thought to protect a person from the plague.

In modern times, in the rare instance when doctors and other medical professionals are faced with a patient with plague, they recommend a treatment that is effective for most people, as long as the disease is caught in time. The standard medical care for plague includes hospitalization and powerful antibiotics, which can kill the harmful bacteria when taken over a number of days. They may be administered intravenously (into the veins), taken orally, or injected in the muscles. It took a multitude of researchers working for more than 100 years to accumulate enough scientific information to make this solution a lifesaving reality.

How You See History

1. If you were an epidemiologist, what questions would you want answered about the spread of the Black Death?
2. How might a rise in plague victims with pneumonic plague have made the transmission of Black Death even worse?
3. Why do you think plague patients agreed to medieval doctors' remedies, even ones that had failed to save others' lives?

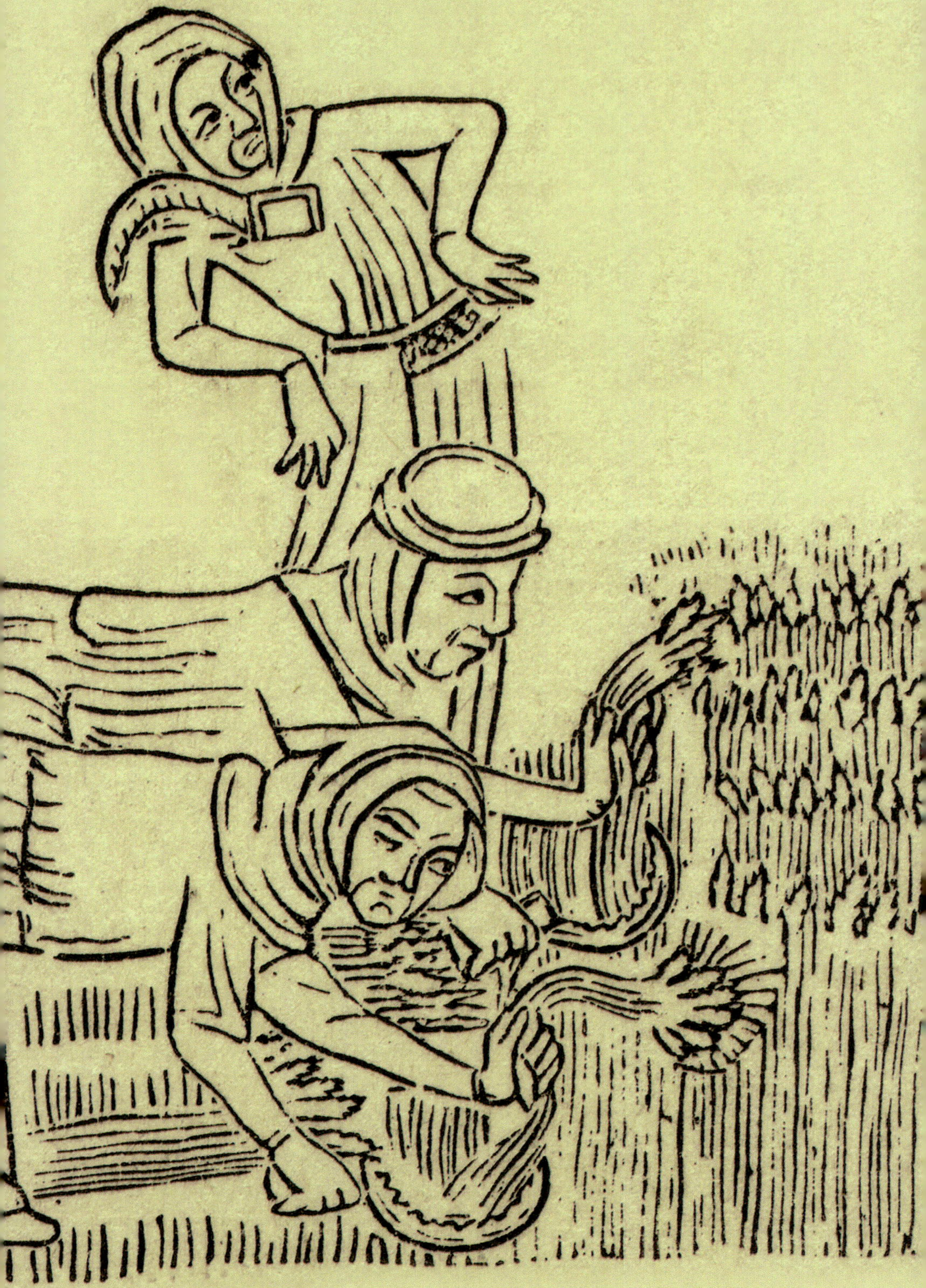

CHAPTER FOUR

A SHIFT IN SOCIETY

Besides the terrible disease itself, the high death toll is often the focus of studies about the Black Death. The plunging drop in population had significant repercussions on the fabric of society in Europe at the time. Life did not return to normal for most people.

The greatest and most immediate changes after the Black Death subsided were economic. Farms were ruined, houses were abandoned, and buildings collapsed without people to repair them. Labor forces were wiped out. Some in the lower classes saw opportunities for social advancement, something that had not been achievable before the plague arrived. They sometimes met with resistance from the ruling upper classes, but the Black Death had unlocked a new era of possibilities. Some historians believe the economic changes after the Black Death ushered in the end of the Middle Ages and the rise of early modern Europe.

The Manorial System Collapses

The biggest single economic change after the Black Death was the decline of the medieval manorial system. This system was based on the manor, which was a large house, and the surrounding lands. These were owned by a wealthy noble or sometimes a knight. The people who worked on a typical manor were called peasants. They

This image of people working in a cornfield was created around 1340, a few years before the Black Death caused much societal upheaval.

FROM THE SOURCE: GUILLAUME DE MACHAUT'S POETRY

Guillaume de Machaut (also spelled Machault) was a French poet and musician during the time of the Black Death. Born around 1300, he worked for royalty for most of his life and was greatly admired for his short poems and musical compositions. In one of his historical poems, Machaut described the effects of depopulation on the large agricultural estates after the Black Death:

For many have certainly
Heard it commonly said
How in one thousand three hundred and forty-nine
Out of one hundred [people] there remained but nine
Thus it happened that for lack of people
Many a splendid farm was left untilled
No one plowed the fields
Bound the cereals [grains] and took in the grapes.[1]

Machaut died in 1377, but his fame spread beyond his home country of France. His work influenced many other writers and musicians.

1. Quoted in David Herlihy, *The Black Death and the Transformation of the West*, ed. Samuel K. Cohn Jr. (Cambridge, MA: Harvard University Press, 1997), p. 41.

owed loyalty to the noble who owned it. Those below his social class generally referred to that owner as "my lord." The lord gave peasants land, a place to live, and protection. In exchange, the peasants labored for him, typically for life. They either worked in the fields, planting and harvesting crops, or did some other form of work.

The vast majority of these laborers were serfs: poor people who were generally attached to the estate on which they lived and worked. Though they were free to leave and look for work somewhere else, if they did so, they no longer had a reliable way to feed their families. Leaving the manor also meant losing the legal and military protection the lord of the manor had provided for them. Afraid that they might not be able to find an equally stable situation elsewhere, most stayed put. They, their children, and their grandchildren remained serfs, providing the cheap labor that made the manorial system possible.

Serfs were the backbone of the manorial system. When millions of those workers suddenly died, that system collapsed. The Black Death killed so many people that entire sections of Europe

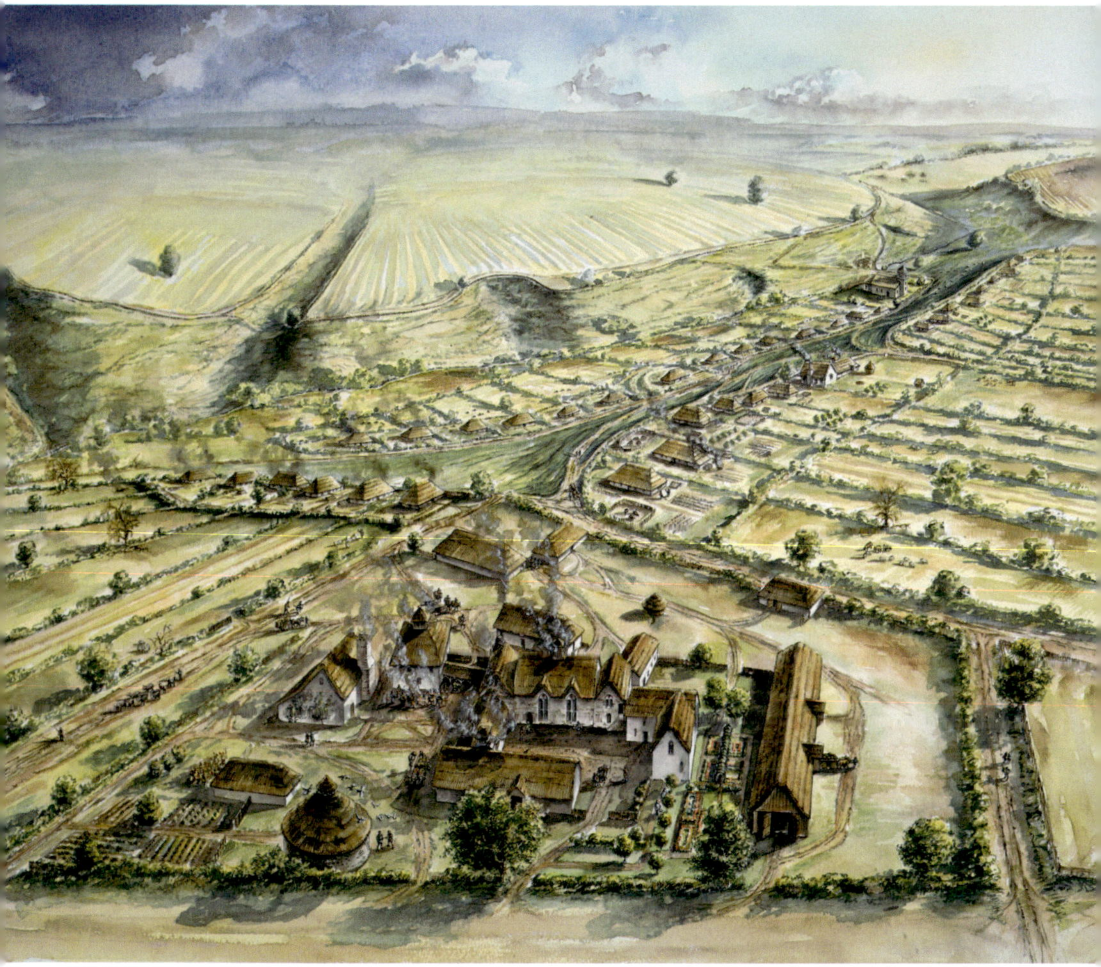

This illustration shows a medieval village, which contained a manor house, smaller houses for peasants, and farmland.

HISTORY HAPPENED HERE: IGHTHAM MOTE

Some manor houses from the time of the Black Death still exist today. One of those is called Ightham (pronounced "item") Mote. Located in Kent, in southeastern England, it is one of the oldest medieval manors in the United Kingdom. The core of the house dates back to the 1340s, the same decade plague was introduced to the country. However, the structure underwent additions and updates in the centuries that followed. A channel of water called a moat surrounds the building, possibly the reason its name includes the word "mote." The house's extensive land includes gardens, an orchard, lakes, and woodland paths.

The last owner of Ightham Mote donated it to the National Trust, an organization that seeks to preserve important historical structures and other parts of cultural heritage in the United Kingdom. Today, people can visit manor houses to learn about their role throughout British history, including the time of the Black Death.

rapidly depopulated. Nearly every manor across Europe suffered terrible losses.

With so much death, many of the nobles who owned manors with extensive agricultural land no longer had enough cheap laborers. They were forced into a difficult position: They could not turn a profit without major changes to their manors. From 1347 to 1353, British lords saw a 20 percent decrease in profits. At the same time, the surviving peasants inhabiting those manors decided to put an added burden on the owners. Many of these serfs realized they suddenly had some bargaining power and demanded a better financial arrangement—an increase in pay.

As a result of these combined factors, the nobles who had long run the manorial system found themselves in an economic crisis. According to historian Robert S. Gottfried:

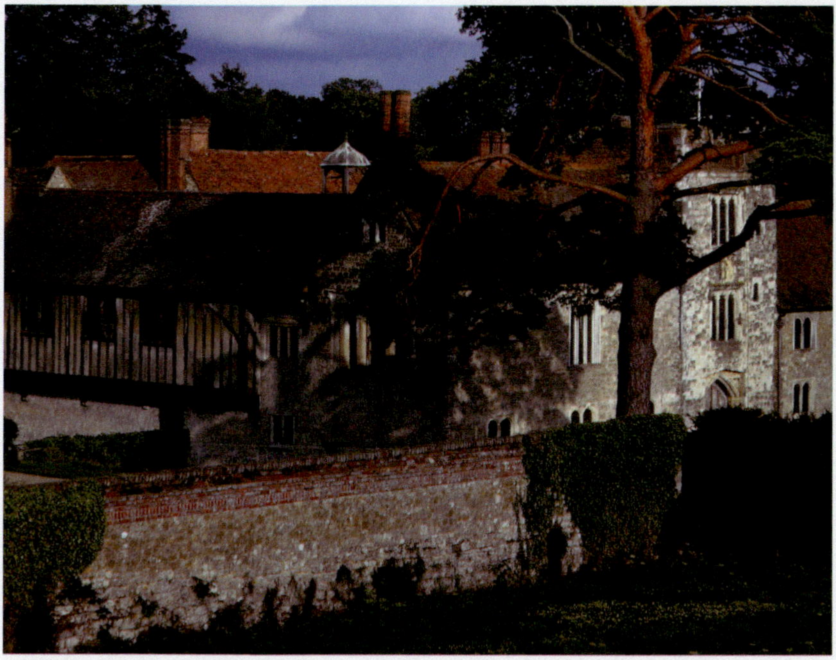

People lived in Ightham Mote for more than 700 years. Today, it exists for education and exploration.

> *The value of agricultural products began to fall, and it stayed low relative to that of industrial goods until the sixteenth century; at the same time, depopulation made agricultural workers scarce and, thus, much more valuable. Wages rose rapidly ... At Cuxham Manor in England, a plowman who was paid 2 shillings a week in 1347 received 7 shillings in 1349, and 10 shillings, 6 pence, by 1350. The result was a dramatic rise in standards of living for those in the lower part of the third order [lower social classes].*[1]

The Lower Class Wants More

Modern scholars and historians base their findings about the Black Death on surviving documents from the era. Several writings of that time describe an upside-down world in which traditional values and wages abruptly underwent massive change. The members of the upper classes found it inappropriate, and even disgraceful, that poorer people began taking advantage of the nobility. Suddenly, these economic demands were coming not only from agricultural laborers but also from commoners in a wide range of jobs in the towns and cities. They wanted higher pay and more benefits, just like their serf counterparts. Furthermore, they were now enjoying goods, services, and customs normally reserved for the wealthy and social elite. In 1363, Italian chronicler Matteo Villani reported:

> *The common folk, both men and women … would no longer labour at their accustomed trades, but demanded the dearest and most delicate [fine] foods for their sustenance; and they married at their will, while children and common women clad themselves in all the fair and costly garments of the [upper-class] ladies dead by that horrible death [plague]. Thus, almost the whole city [Florence], without any restraint whatsoever, rushed into disorderliness of life … Men dreamed of wealth and abundance in garments and in all other things … [and] the work of all trades and crafts rose in disorderly fashion beyond the double.*[2]

It was not only the traditionally poor classes that took advantage of the widespread death. Skilled professionals, especially doctors, suffered terrible losses during the Black Death. Because these professionals had to be in close contact with the plague's victims, very few were willing to step up to replace them. The replacements were able to charge premium prices for their services simply because they were the only ones who would do them. The clergy was also hit particularly hard, resulting in fewer priests and chaplains. Some churches were left without clergy. Many surviving clergy refused to continue their service without higher salaries.

Keeping the Classes Separate

The significant increase in salaries was not the only example of rising prices in the years following the Black Death. Because so many people, including artisans and other skilled workers, had died during

THEY MADE HISTORY: IBN KHALDŪN

The major economic cost of the Black Death was not restricted to Europe. A Muslim Arab scholar—Ibn Khaldūn—wrote about that time, providing an account of the extensive devastation to the Islamic regions of the Middle East and North Africa.

Ibn Khaldūn was born in North Africa in 1332. Both of his parents died during the Black Death. He held government jobs for much of life but decided to retire and write history books. In his most well-known book, the *Muqaddimah*, he described the Black Death:

> *Civilization both in the East and the West was visited by a destructive plague which devastated nations and caused populations to vanish. It swallowed up many of the good things of civilization and wiped them out ... Cities and buildings were laid waste, roads and way signs were obliterated, settlements and mansions became empty, dynasties [family lines of rulers] and tribes grew weak. The entire inhabited world changed ... It was as if the voice of existence in the world had called out for oblivion and restriction, and the world responded to its call.*[1]

Ibn Khaldūn became a teacher and judge later in life. He died in Cairo, Egypt, in 1406.

1. Quoted in Michael Dols, *The Black Death in the Middle East* (Princeton, NJ: Princeton University Press, 1977), p. 67.

the epidemic, very few people were left to produce everyday goods. These included food, wine, fabrics, clothing, linens, pottery, metal utensils and weapons, building materials, and more. The production of fewer goods made those goods more valuable. This contributed to a general rise in the prices of goods and services throughout society, which is known as inflation. This inflation "persisted until the last decades of the fourteenth century," historian David Herlihy wrote. This meant "that under the shock of [the] plague, production in town and countryside had fallen even more rapidly than the population."[3]

Most of the nobles and other wealthy people could afford to pay the higher prices, of course, although they were certainly unhappy about it. Before the plague, there was no way that most members of the lower classes could afford to pay the inflated prices. However, because of the plague, large numbers of these workers had demanded and were now making more money. As Villani pointed out, many people who were not used to luxuries now ate fine foods and wore expensive garments. The peasants undoubtedly appreciated this change in lifestyle. However, the upper classes, who were used to being the only people who could enjoy luxury, hated this trend. They were angry to see people they viewed as inferiors enjoying access to fine goods.

Hoping to keep the class system clearly divided, the nobles who ran the governments across Europe passed hundreds of laws regulating how people could spend money in the century following the Black Death. These were restrictions designed to limit displays of wealth. For instance, women were forbidden to wear dresses that did not conform to a certain style, and only certain types of food and drink could be served at weddings.

These laws were written so that they applied to members of the lower classes but not to aristocratic people. The obvious goal was reinforcement of the boundaries between the social classes. Unfortunately for the upper classes, they did not work. The higher living standards of many commoners in the post-plague years remained a fact of life for the remainder of the medieval era.

Controlling Commoners

In desperation, a few national rulers and town governments tried to keep the lower social groups in their place by more obvious and forceful means. Some rules forbade peasants from leaving the manors on which they had been raised. Others kept commoners who

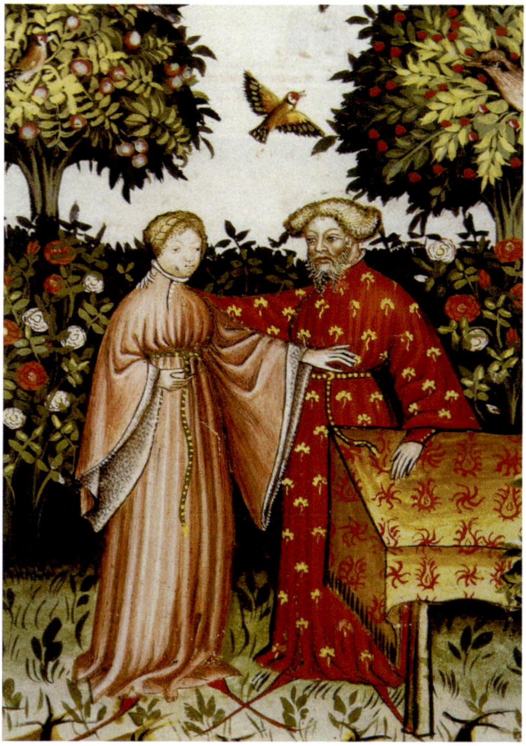

Because of restrictions on what members of the lower classes wore, there was a clearly visible distinction between members of the upper classes, shown here, and so-called commoners.

worked in shops and other businesses from switching jobs. Still others placed limits on how much commoners could earn in various jobs and professions. As scholar Philip Ziegler explained, the object of these rules

> *was to pin wages and prices as closely as possible to a pre-plague figure and thus to check the inflation that existed in the England of 1349-51. The Government realised that this could never be achieved so long as labourers were free to move from one employer to another in search of higher wages and so long as employers were free to woo away labourers from their neighbours with advantageous offers. By restricting the right of an employee to leave his place of work, by compelling him to accept work when it was offered to him, by forbidding the employer to offer wages greater than those paid three years before … [and] by fixing the prices which butchers, bakers and fishmongers could charge their customers, they hoped to re-create the conditions that pertained [existed] before the plague and maintain them for ever.*[4]

Any citizen who ignored these oppressive rules was taxed or fined, and some who refused to pay the fines were arrested. Such

PAST MEETS PRESENT: THE MODERN CLASS SYSTEM

As the structure of society changed in the Middle Ages, different systems replaced the rigid groupings of the medieval manorial system. In modern times, for example, the United States, Canada, and many other countries have a class system. Classes are not based in law, however, but have more to do with wealth.

The class groups are mainly divided into upper, middle, and lower classes, though many social scientists include smaller groups within these. The upper class owns most of the wealth and has control over large businesses. Some in this group have inherited their wealth, while others earned it. Just a small percentage of people belong to this group. The remainder of a population is split between the middle class and lower class. Generally, people can move between the classes, depending on how much money they earn. However, social conditions can make it difficult to break into a higher class. For example, those of the upper and middle classes often can attain a higher education, which opens them up to higher paying careers. Those in the lower class may not have the financial means to attend colleges and universities. So, while the class systems of today are more flexible than those of medieval times, obstacles to social mobility remain.

extreme measures ended up affecting everyone except society's wealthiest members and, as such, were very unpopular. Attempts to regulate wages and maintain the old social order only made peasants angry. The result was a series of uprisings by workers that foreshadowed the larger anti-aristocratic revolutions that would rock Europe in the 1700s and 1800s. Probably the best-known example in the 14th century occurred in France in 1358. Because French peasants were often called "Jacques," it was called the Jacquerie. The French chronicler Jean Froissart recorded the following:

Thus they [a large number of peasants] gathered together without any other counsel [leaders], and without any armour saving [except for] staves [sticks] and knives, and so went to the house of a knight dwelling thereby, and brake [broke] up his house and slew the knight and the lady and all his children great and small and brent [burned] his house. And they then went to another castle, and took the knight thereof and bound him fast to a stake, and then … slew the lady and his daughter and all his other children, and then slew the knight by great torment and burnt and beat down the castle. And so they did to divers [many] other castles and good houses; and they multiplied so that they were a six thousand [rebels], and ever as they went forward they increased [in number] … so that every gentleman fled from them and took their wives and children with them … and left their house void and their goods therein. These mischievous people thus assembled without captain … robbed, brent [burned], and slew all gentlemen that they could lay hands on.[5]

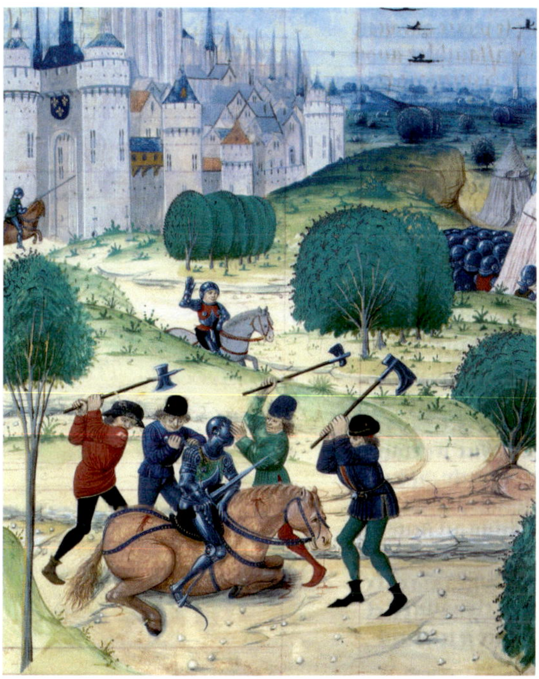

This is an illustration of Jean Froissart's account of a peasants' revolt in France. It shows peasants attacking a knight. A knight would have occupied a high place in society, acquiring wealth and land through military service to a lord or king.

These violent acts were an expression of the anger that had been building up in peasants for generations. After the plague, they had finally gotten a taste of a better life, and just like the nobles, they were unwilling to give it up without a fight. These feelings were not unique

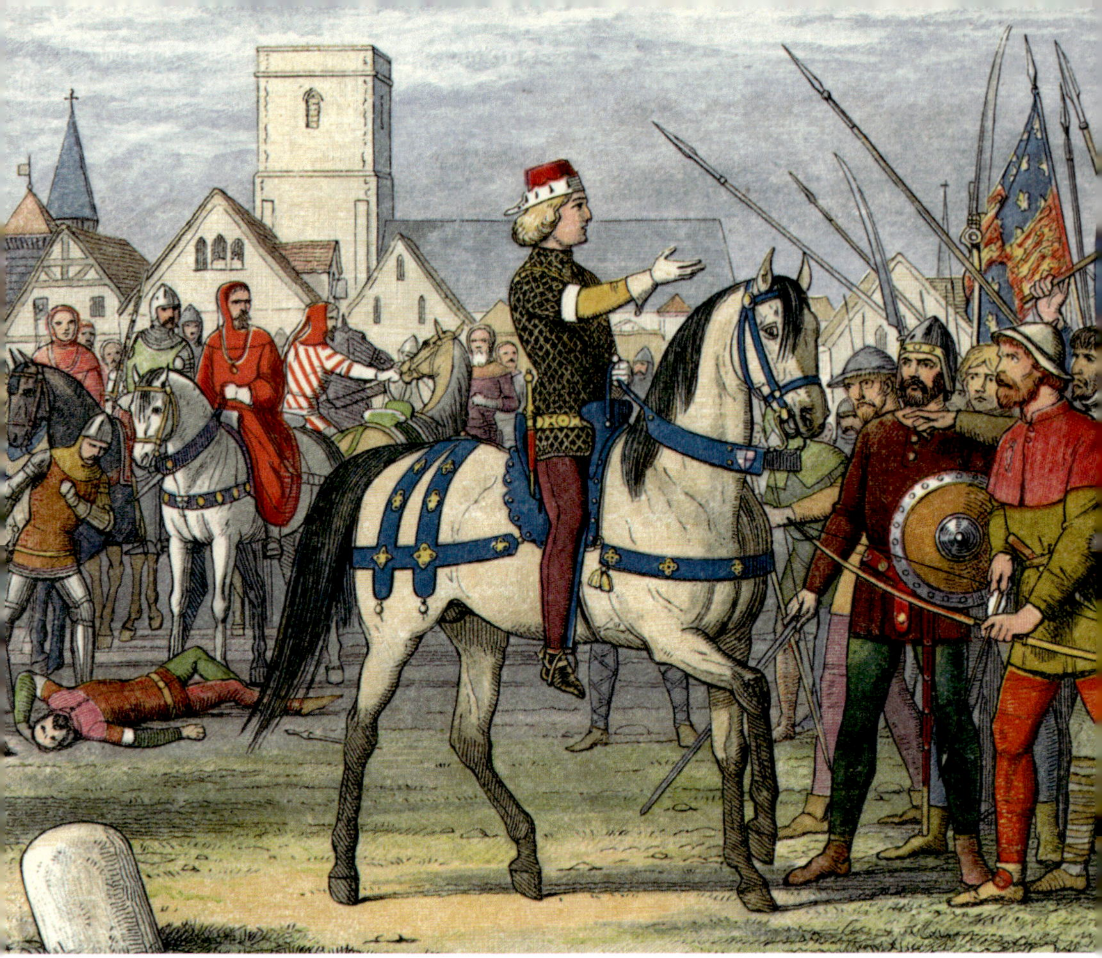

In this artist's look at the Peasants' Revolt in England of 1381, King Richard II tries to make peace with rebelling peasants. The man lying dead on the ground was the leader of the rebellion, Wat Tyler.

to the French. A similarly large peasant revolt occurred in England in 1381. There, King Richard II felt so threatened that he came to a legal agreement with the peasants, granting them a number of rights and freedoms they had never before possessed. Although the king and his nobles did not end up honoring the full agreement, England's lower classes did gain some rights by compromising with King Richard. The government had to reduce taxes, and it was not permitted to pass any laws designed to keep the wages of ordinary laborers low. As a result of these substantial changes, England's traditional manorial system had vanished from most parts of the kingdom by the early 15th century.

Evaporating Upper Class

The Black Death turned the fortunes of many survivors upside down. While some upper-class landowners took the opportunity to add the lands of deceased property owners to their holdings, those in the lower classes, too, had the chance to buy up land since there was less competition for it. However, many rich people found their fortunes reduced after the plague had died down. They had relied on serfs to farm their lands and produce food and goods. When so many peasants died of plague, the source of income on many large estates greatly decreased or dried up completely.

As a consequence of the Black Death, many peasant land plots were abandoned. Those peasants who survived were often able to reduce their obligations to the landowner because the landowner had fewer peasants working for him. In short, peasants were in high demand. Some landowners became impoverished because of the loss of labor and the decline of the purchasing power of their money. The Black Death had created an economic situation in which some of the wealthy became poorer and some of the poor became wealthier. It would continue to have implications for many other aspects of European culture as well.

How You See History

1. Why do you think the upper classes were so resistant to raising wages for laborers?
2. Why did laws and regulations fail to stop the breakdown of the medieval manorial system?
3. Do you think the changes to medieval society would have happened without the Black Death? Why or why not?

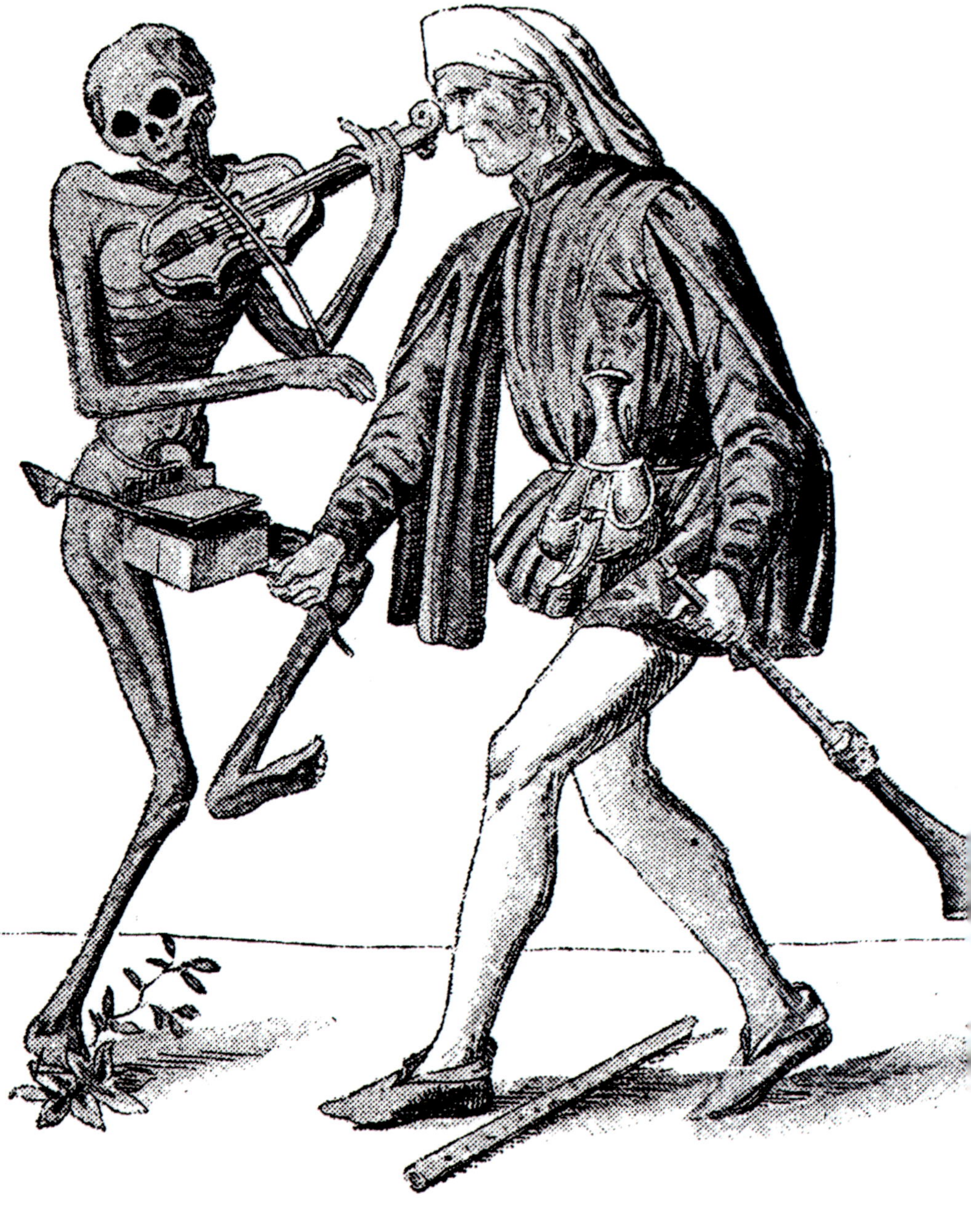

CHAPTER FIVE

CULTURAL CONSEQUENCES

While economic and societal changes were among the most obvious adjustments in the post–Black Death world, they were hardly the only areas affected. The immense pressure of living with so much death and disease irrevocably altered nearly every aspect of European culture imaginable. Changes in art, religion, medicine, technology, and education around this time can clearly be traced to the Black Death. People even began behaving differently, according to some eyewitness accounts, and this change in behavior was most often for the worse.

Bad Behaviors

Some of the most visible aspects of life that changed after the Black Death were general behaviors and relationships. However, many of the worst examples were merely temporary. For instance, Boccaccio described various episodes of antisocial behavior that occurred at the height of the Black Death. These included brothers abandoning brothers, priests fleeing their churches, and parents neglecting their children. However, later observers pointed out that these shameful acts were part of the mass hysteria created by the immediate danger of horrible illness and death. As a result, these behaviors were

Death always seemed to be "dancing" around the survivors of the Black Death, and the cultural trends of the period reflected this theme.

widespread but only short-term. After the great outbreak of pestilence ran its course, such extreme reactions were less common.

Still, some of Boccaccio's peers wrote about other, more long-term negative changes in the following years. French monk and chronicler Jean de Venette said that a number of people displayed thoughtless and selfish behavior:

> *After the cessation [end] of the epidemic, pestilence, or plague, the men and women who survived married each other ... Pregnant women were seen on every side ... But woe is me! the world was not changed for the better but for the worse by this renewal of population. For men were more avaricious and grasping [greedy] than before, even though they had far greater possessions. They were more covetous and disturbed each other more frequently with [law]suits, brawls, [and] disputes ... The enemies of the king of France and of the Church were stronger and wickeder than before and stirred up wars on sea and on land. Greater evils than before pullulated [spread] everywhere in the world.*[1]

It is difficult to know how much of this description is based on changes that affected the entire continent and how much reflected mainly de Venette's personal experiences. Regardless, evidence does conclusively show that life did not go back to normal after the Black Death. As soon as fear of plague began to subside, several more outbreaks struck Europe in the second half of the century. Although smaller than the initial epidemic, these new threats discouraged many people and forced them to view life as uncertain and brutal. The possibility of dying from an unpreventable disease or facing turbulent economic change made 14th-century and 15th-century Europe unstable.

The Dance of Death

Some experts speculate that many people began to have a more gruesome way of looking at the concepts of life and death. While everyone hoped for a long and successful life, most people now recognized how easily death could come to anyone. Because of the periodic outbreaks of plague and the huge numbers of dead that

HISTORY HAPPENED HERE: THE FRESCOES OF ST. MARY OF THE ROCKS

The Sanctuary of St. Mary of the Rocks, located just outside the village of Beram in Croatia, holds treasured art from the time after the Black Death. The church's walls are covered with frescoes created by artist Vincent de Kastav in the 1400s. Frescoes are wall or ceiling paintings completed on wet plaster with watercolors. Kastav painted scenes from the New Testament of the Bible as well as his famous *Dance of Death*, completed in 1474.

In the *Dance of Death*, skeletons representing death lead deceased people out of the land of the living into the realm of the dead. The dead include people young and old, rich and poor, of all professions and backgrounds, demonstrating that death comes for everyone.

St. Mary of the Rocks is usually closed to protect the invaluable artwork inside, but visitors are welcome. A villager holds a key and escorts people to the church, which is located in a forest.

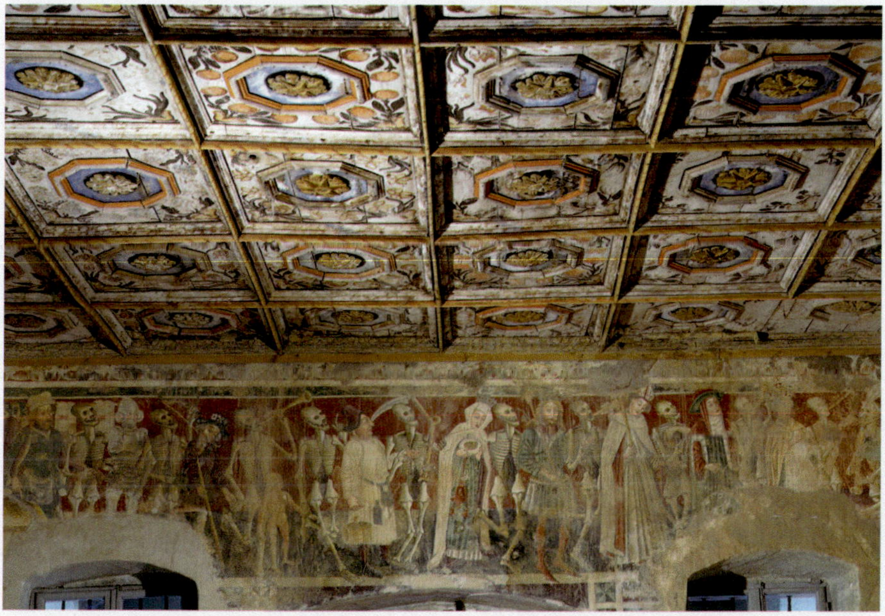

Vincent de Kastav's fresco reflects the danse macabre, or dance of death, theme that was prevalent after the time of the Black Death.

FROM THE SOURCE: "EVERYWHERE IS FEAR"

The onset of the Black Death inspired many Europeans to express their horror or sadness in writing. Some of these writings have come to be seen as pieces of literary art. An outstanding example was written by the Italian author Petrarch. Petrarch (born Francesco Petrarca) was one of the most important scholars of that time, a mentor to Boccaccio, and a founder of the movement called humanism. Humanism ushered in the cultural movement called the Renaissance, which marked the end of the Middle Ages.

In this letter to his brother, a monk, Petrarch talks about the devastating consequences of the Black Death:

> *Alas! my beloved brother, what shall I say? How shall I begin? Whither [where] shall I turn? On all sides is sorrow; everywhere is fear. I would [wish], my brother, that I had never been born, or, at least, had died before these times. How will posterity believe that there has been a time when without the lightnings of heaven or the fires of earth, without wars or other visible slaughter, not*

came with them, the end of life was always right around the corner. The most common image of this new outlook was the macabre, a style that used skeletons and other images of death as a centerpiece. Artists, sculptors, and writers all frequently used this new and popular style. Often, they showed or described one or more skeletons dancing, a frightening theme that is known as the danse macabre, or dance of death.

A widespread fascination with that chilling image spread all across Europe in the late 14th and early 15th centuries. It was not just the loss of loved ones to plague that motivated this obsession with dark and terrifying art. Rather, it was also the fear of one's own death, which they believed could come without warning.

this or that part of the earth, but well-nigh [nearly] the whole globe, has remained without inhabitants. When has any such thing been even heard or seen; in what annals [histories] has it ever been read that houses were left vacant, cities deserted, the country neglected, the fields too small for the dead and a fearful and universal solitude over the whole earth?[1]

1. Quoted in "Petrarch on the Plague," Decameron Web, modified February 18, 2010, www.brown.edu/Departments/Italian_Studies/dweb/plague/perspectives/petrarca.php.

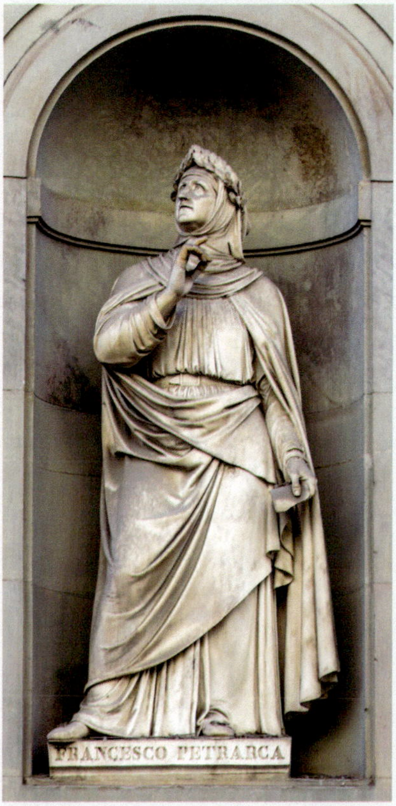

This statue of poet and scholar Petrarch is found in Florence, Italy.

The dance of death and other dark, pessimistic images were part of the larger view of a changed world. The general agreement in the post-plague years was that the traditional order of the universe had gone wrong. Some people argued that God had spread so much death because he was angry about human sins. However, many others believed that the disaster was too big to be explained by God alone. There had to be some other factor, one that was perhaps beyond human understanding.

The Matter of Faith

The way that most Europeans viewed death, God, and life in general had been permanently altered. One of the leading modern experts on the Black Death, Philip Ziegler, called it "a crisis of faith," arguing that

> *assumptions which had been taken for granted for centuries were now in question, the very framework of men's reasoning seemed to be breaking up. And though the Black Death was far from being the only cause, the anguish and disruption which it had inflicted made the greatest single contribution to the disintegration of an age.*[2]

In Europe, the Roman Catholic Church was by far the largest spiritual institution during the Middle Ages. People looked to the Church and clergymen for guidance in every part of their lives. However, the Black Death caused millions of devoted Catholics to begin questioning their trust in priests, their relationship to God, and the pope himself.

Many Europeans in the 14th century were unsure of God's role in the spread of plague because they believed God was invisible and did not communicate with people. On the other hand, members of the clergy were visible, and their behavior during the crisis was well known. Many priests and bishops died of plague, so it was clear that even a close relationship to God could not save someone from the disease. Some saw this as a strike against them. Many people also felt that the clergy had no ability to persuade God to stop illness or spare the millions who died. Worst of all, however, was that many priests had simply abandoned their posts, leaving the people who put their faith in them to suffer and die, thinking that God had abandoned them.

Despite many leaving their posts, nearly 50 percent of clergy across Europe lost their lives to plague. The central Church authorities needed to quickly replace as many of them as they could. Training programs in universities and on-the-job training were accelerated so that the new priests could start their jobs immediately. While these methods were effective in producing new clergy members, the priests were commonly regarded as being much worse than those who came before them. Some reports claimed that they were often not even literate, which was one of the greatest distinctions between common people and the clergy before the Black Death.

In addition, people felt that Pope Clement VI in Avignon, France, had not set a good example during the catastrophe. Rumors spread

Clergy and others pray for relief from plague in this depiction of the Black Death period.

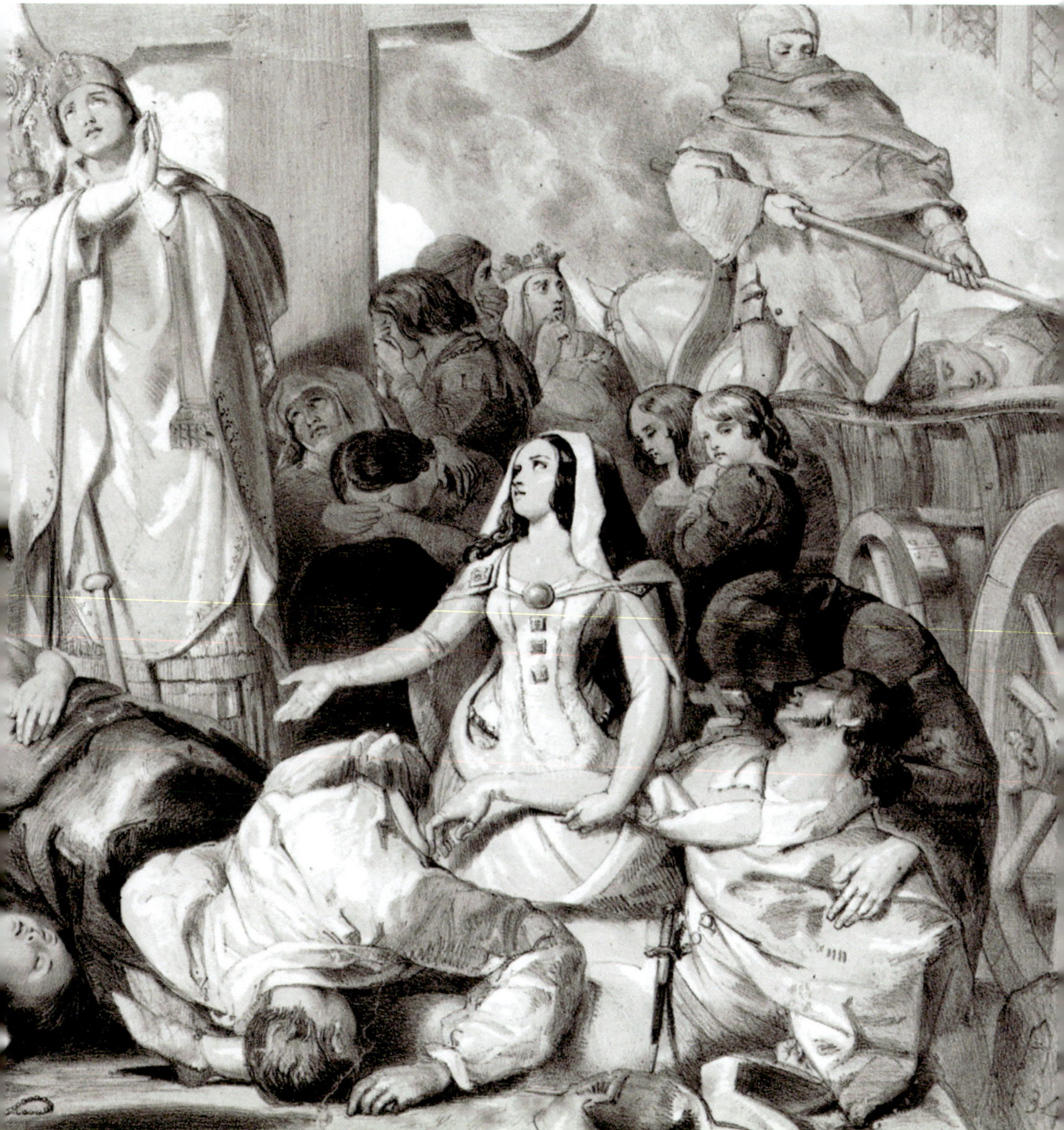

that instead of risking his life to help his followers, he went to extreme lengths to save himself.

The Church's high place in society sustained a major blow. Following the outbreak of the Black Death, most Europeans continued to believe in God, and while some left the Catholic Church, many decided to stay. Those who remained now felt that priests were not necessarily the special individuals that most people had previously assumed they were. More shockingly, almost everyone now believed that the Church had flaws. Although the Church remained a powerful social institution, scholar James C. Giblin pointed out that

> *it never regained the complete authority it had enjoyed before the plague. Once people began to question the Church's actions, they kept on questioning them. This eventually led to attempts to reform the Roman Catholic Church and then, in the sixteenth century, to the establishment of the first Protestant churches.*[3]

Many of the daily and yearly religious habits and traditions of Europeans began to change as the Church fell from its place of highest esteem. Before the plague, it was an everyday event for someone who felt troubled, worried, or lost to ask their local clergyman to pray for him or her. However, in the post-plague era, it became increasingly common for people to ask their loved ones to do so or to pray for themselves instead.

Interestingly, near the end of the Black Death, Europe witnessed a major increase in charitable giving. Hospitals, the poor, and others in need of public support benefited from the increase in good works by the faithful. In addition, large numbers of people left their normal activities and went on long, difficult pilgrimages to holy Christian sites. Among the most popular were the church in Canterbury, England, where Saint Thomas Becket had been murdered; the sites of Jesus's arrest, trial, and crucifixion in Jerusalem; Saint Peter's tomb in Rome; and Santiago de Compostela, a city in Spain where the shrine of Saint James is located.

Many scholars think that the increased religious offerings during this time period were believed to be a way to make peace with God.

Those who still believed in God hoped this would persuade God to not send any more destructive plagues to punish humanity.

Turning to Technology

Science and knowledge in general were other important aspects of culture affected by the Black Death. The technological advances during the years after the plague are particularly important. Before plague began spreading in the mid-1300s, most unskilled labor was accomplished by hand or with the aid of some simple tools. However, when a large number of Europe's workers died in the epidemic, there were no longer enough hands to do all the work that needed to be done.

Solutions to this major problem needed to be found—and found fast. One obvious fix was to produce more tools that could make work easier. As a result, there were significant developments in the most basic necessity for farming: plows. Their improvement allowed farmers to accomplish more work in less time. However, simply improving old tools would not be enough. New kinds of devices were needed.

One example of an advance was related to the European fishing industry. Before the Black Death, fishermen routinely came ashore to salt the fish they had recently caught, which would preserve them for a long time. Then, they sailed back out and caught more fish. Just like in the rest of the economy, this process no longer had enough people to keep it up, so the number of fish that could be caught and preserved was too small to sustain people's needs. Trying to find solutions to this problem, in the late 1300s, Dutch fishermen found a way of salting, drying, and storing their catch aboard their vessels.

One of the most important and influential technological advances of all time also occurred during this post-plague period: the invention of the improved printing press. This printing press with movable type immediately revolutionized the production, distribution, and consumption of literature and other written materials. Indeed, few inventions in history have transformed the world as much as this one. Before movable type, the only way to produce a book was to write it by hand; these kinds of books are known as manuscripts. The manuscript then had to be very carefully copied by hand over and over again. Before the Black Death, this job was done by thousands of highly trained individuals called copyists. Bookmakers in Europe were left without a strong workforce after the plague, but the demand for books was higher than ever. Historian David Herlihy explained:

> *The late medieval population plunge raised labor costs and also raised the premium to be claimed by the one who could devise a cheaper way of reproducing books. Johann Gutenberg's invention of printing on the basis of movable metal type in 1453 was only the culmination [result] of many experiments carried on across the previous century. His genius was in finding a way to combine several technologies into the new art.*[4]

The Black Death also improved medical knowledge and techniques during the late 14th century. People were painfully aware that their doctors had not had the knowledge or ability to stop plague. Later outbreaks of the disease in the 1390s and early 1400s only reinforced the need for advances in medical science.

Many European doctors took their failures seriously and admitted they did not know enough about the human body. To fix this shortcoming, Pope Clement VI reversed the Church's law regarding the dissection of dead humans. Called cadavers, dead human bodies had been off-limits for educational purposes for a long time. Studying cadavers brought about major new advances in the emerging science of anatomy, which is the study of the human body. There was also a new interest and confidence in direct surgical methods. European universities rarely taught surgery in the pre-plague years, but some began adding surgical instruction in the century following the Black Death.

Effects on Education

Education in Europe changed after the Black Death, just like so many other spheres of life. One factor driving that change was that many teachers had died. Scholars and teachers tended to be older, and older people were more vulnerable to the disease. In fact,

THEY MADE HISTORY: JOHANNES GUTENBERG

Although often incorrectly noted as the inventor of the printing press, German craftsman Johannes Gutenberg was actually—just as importantly—the first to make and use a practical movable type printing press. Movable type means blocks with raised letters or other characters that can be arranged and rearranged to print words. These blocks made it much easier and faster to print books and other materials. Movable type was used for the next 500 years.

Born around 1395, Johannes Gutenberg (born Johann Gensfleisch zur Laden zum Gutenberg) was born in Mainz, Germany. He became a talented metalworker and began to experiment with metal and wood type in combination with presses for making wine and paper. Gutenberg used his newly created printing press in around 1455 to complete what is now called the Gutenberg Bible. He lost his print shop to a lawsuit soon after, but he likely opened another one. Gutenberg died in Mainz in 1468.

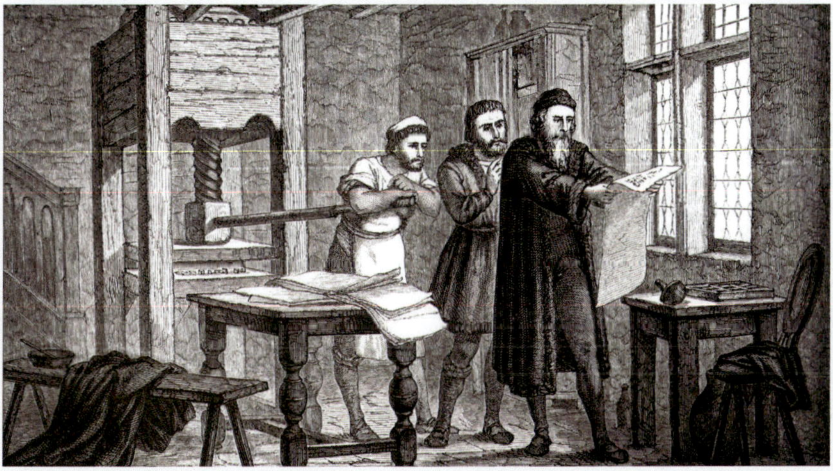

Though the Chinese actually invented movable type about 400 years before Gutenberg's press, the German inventor Johannes Gutenberg introduced the technology to the West.

PAST MEETS PRESENT: HUMAN DISSECTION

Without being able to dissect a human body that had been stricken with plague, it was hard for medieval doctors and scientists to see the effects the disease had on the inside of the body. Dissections allowed medicine to advance.

The dissection of cadavers is still of paramount importance in the field of medicine. Almost every medical student dissects a human body. To them, it is the best way to experience the body's intricacy. Even if the students do not become surgeons, they can get a sense of the parts of the body at work through dissection. Cadavers also allow doctors to practice procedures before performing them on living people who can feel pain. Not all cadavers are used to teach, though most are. Others are used by car companies to study the effects of crashes on human bodies in order to improve safety standards. Still others are used by drug companies and private organizations.

In the United States, people must agree to donate their body for research. Bodies cannot be bought or sold. Each year, an estimated 20,000 Americans donate their body for scientific research.

several known European universities seem to have disappeared in the mid-1300s. A sharp decline in both instructors and students due to plague deaths is a likely reason. So, the need for more educated members of society was obvious. New colleges and universities began to fulfill this role, such as Trinity Hall in Cambridge, England, established in 1350.

Modern scholars also point out that the decline of Latin as the language of learning was tied to the Black Death. This change opened up learning to more people, who could read and study in their own language rather than having to learn Latin first, as many teachers and priests had to do previously. Historian

William H. McNeill explained that "the decay of Latin as a *lingua franca* [shared language] among the educated men of Western Europe was hastened by the die-off of clerics and teachers who knew enough Latin to keep that ancient tongue alive."[5] The less frequent use of Latin and the increased access to literature, thanks to the movable type printing press, made knowledge more accessible to all. In just a few years, the Black Death had altered the course of education—and life—for everyone in Europe.

How You See History

1. Why do you think the skeletons are dancing in the plague-inspired theme called the danse macabre, or dance of death?
2. How did the development of Gutenberg's printing press promote literacy among different classes of people?
3. Do you think advances would have been made in medicine, education, and other areas without the Black Death? Why or why not?

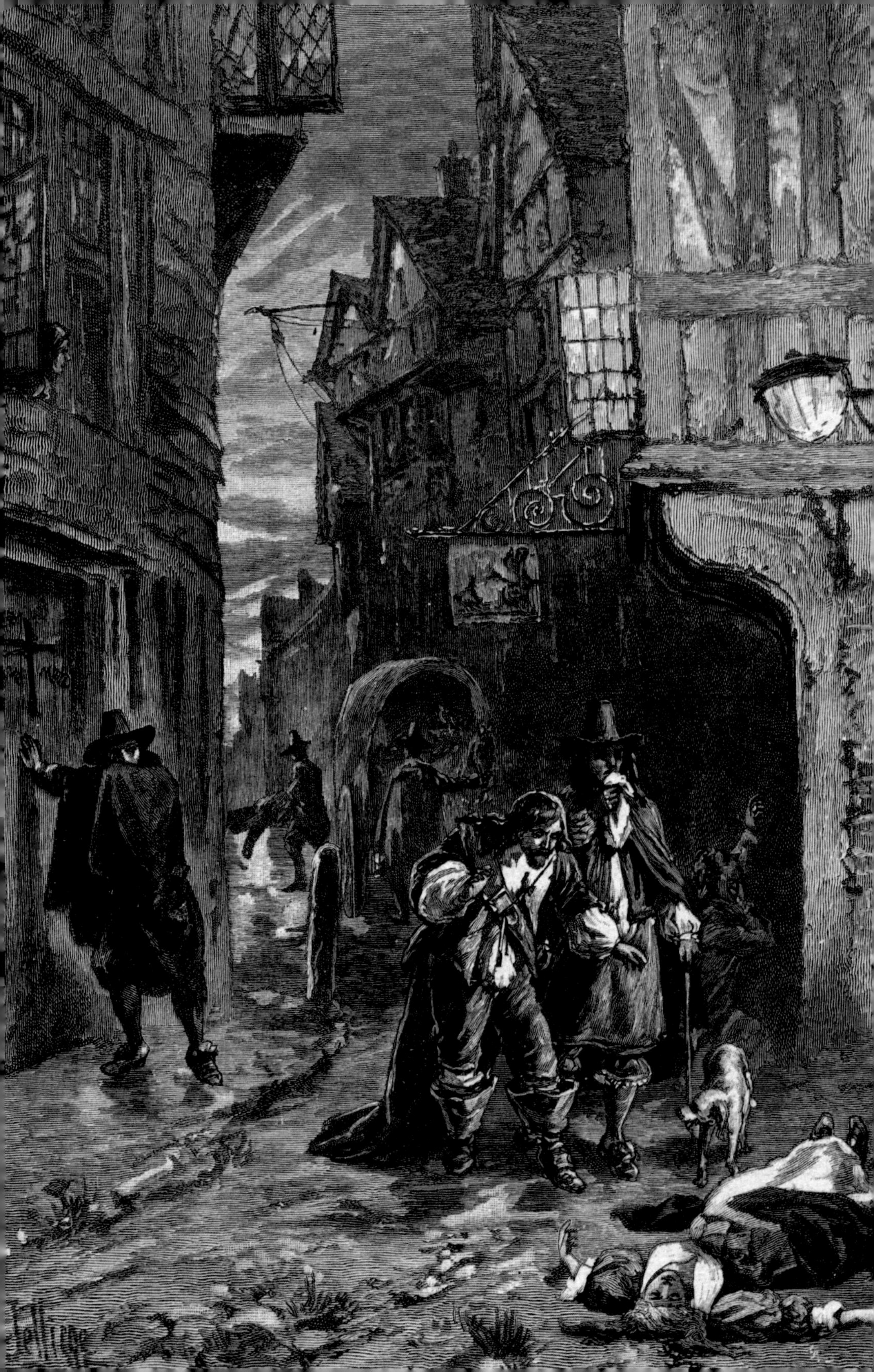

CHAPTER SIX

THE REAPPEARING PLAGUE

The Black Death had largely ended in most places by 1351. However, the destruction it left behind was nearly beyond belief. For example, Florence, Italy, lost about 50,000 people out of its total population of 85,000. Many modern researchers think about 30 percent of Europe's overall population died from plague, but it may have been closer to 50 percent, according to a few sources. Life for those remaining was forever changed.

Unfortunately, the terrible disease did not disappear entirely. It returned a number of times. Although no reappearance was as devastating as the Black Death, each took an awful toll, killing thousands, spreading terror, and shaking economies. The population of Europe did not return to pre–Black Death numbers until around 1550.

Medical science's advances in the early modern era provided a basic understanding that most diseases are caused by germs, including the bacterium responsible for the Black Death. Although *Yersinia pestis* still exists, it no longer poses the terrible threat to individuals that it once did. Today, very few people outside of Africa and a few other places need to worry about plague. It has not been forgotten,

After the Black Death, the worst occurrence of plague in London began in 1665 and is depicted here. More than 68,000 deaths were recorded, but historians think the actual number was likely more than 100,000.

however. The Black Death remains a dark reminder of the horrors of a pandemic.

Coming Back

The plague outbreaks that struck Europe in the centuries immediately following the Black Death continued to be frightening and destructive. People were still in the dark about the cause, how it spread, and effective ways to treat those who contracted the disease.

The first major reappearance of the disease after 1351 was a decade later. In 1361, the *pestis secunda* (second plague) arrived in Europe. "The return of plague was a nightmare reborn," historian Robert Gottfried wrote. He added:

> *While primarily an attack of bubonic plague and not as severe as the Black Death, the* pestis secunda *was still one of the most lethal epidemics in history. Many observers … believed it was especially deadly for select groups, including the young.*[1]

So many young people died during the plague of 1361 that it was nicknamed "the children's plague." It is possible the reason for this was that children under 10 years old did not have any immunity to resist the disease, whereas those who had lived through the Black Death had acquired some immunity. Based on historical research, it is estimated that 10 to 20 percent of Europe's entire population was killed in the second arrival of plague.

After that, the plague seemed to just keep returning. Every few years, it reappeared, sometimes in one country, other times in several, forming a kind of plague cycle. England, for instance, had significant outbreaks in 1369, 1379 to 1383, 1390 to 1391, 1405 to 1406, 1411 to 1412, 1426 to 1429, and several other times in the three centuries that followed.

Although none of these outbreaks reproduced the gigantic death toll of the Black Death, the suffering of families and victims was no less intense. During a 1471 outbreak in England, a man visiting London sent a letter to his relatives in Norfolk. He wrote, "I pray you send me word if any of our friends or well-willers

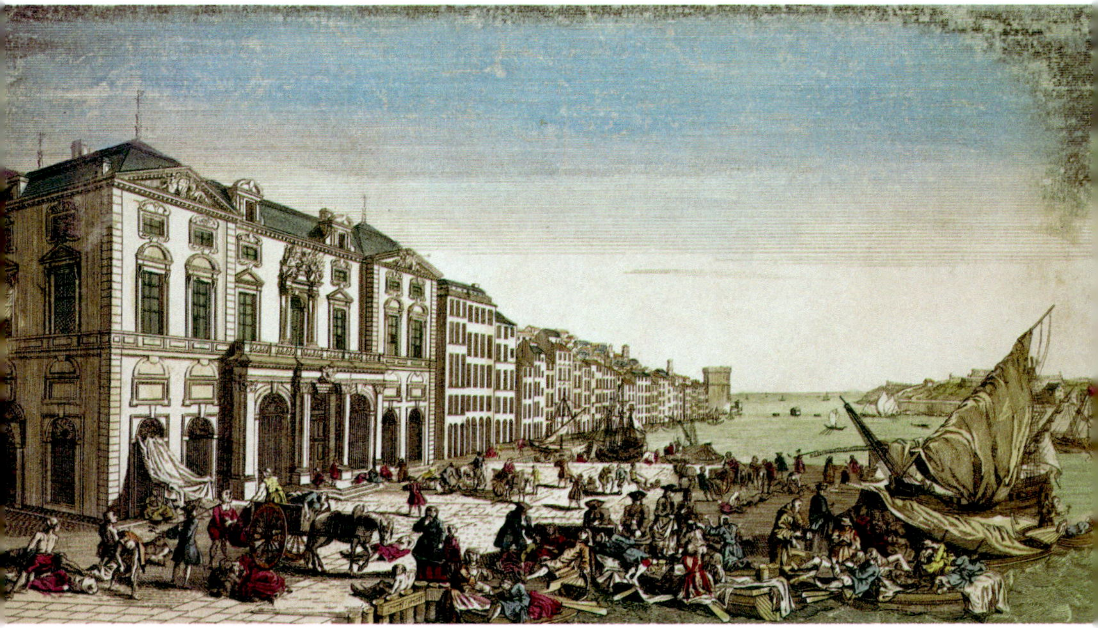

The last major outbreak of plague in Europe happened in Marseille, France, in 1720, depicted here. It killed more than 100,000 people.

be dead, for I fear that there is great death … in Norfolk; for I ensure you, it is the most universal death that ever I [witnessed] in England."[2]

The horror of this seemingly endless cycle of plague and death in Europe can be seen in various surviving statistics. As an example, one region of northern Germany, Thurungia, had 179 villages in 1300, before the first onset of plague. In 1500, after numerous outbreaks of the disease in the region, only 33 of those villages still existed. The rest had been abandoned, wiped out by plague and its effects.

Major outbreaks of bubonic plague eventually slowed, and the disease became considerably less lethal. Over time, people developed some precautions against it. In the early 1700s in what is now Hungary, for example, hundreds of checkpoints were set up and manned by thousands of guards. These acted as quarantine walls by limiting traders and other human traffic moving into Europe from the East.

Pasteur's Discoveries

The most important factors in humanity's victory over plague are the 19th-century discovery that germs cause disease and the later identification of the specific bacterium that causes plague. When combined with better health practices in much of Europe in the 1800s, scientific knowledge helped minimize the death toll from many harmful diseases, including plague.

The key period during which many of these breakthroughs were made began in 1854. That year, French scientist Louis Pasteur successfully demonstrated that germs cause certain foods to change their chemical composition. Scientists were aware of the existence of germs before that, but they had assumed that these tiny organisms played no major role in nature. In his experiments, Pasteur showed that they had been invisible but active throughout history. Next, Pasteur and some other scientists set out to confirm something they already suspected—that germs not only cause disease but can protect against it as well.

Pasteur found his proof by chance. He was studying cholera, a deadly disease common in chickens and other birds, and he had to obtain some samples of the germs and use them for experiments. Every two weeks, he would inject cholera bacteria into his laboratory animals, allow them to get sick, and then extract the germs again. This ensured that his supply of germs was always fresh and strong. After he went on vacation and let one batch of bacteria sit for more than a month, he tried to circulate it and get some new samples. However, sitting on a lab table for so long had weakened the cholera germs; they did not cause an infection. Confused, Pasteur continued investigating why this occurred. Eventually, he discovered that if a very weak group of disease-causing bacteria is introduced to an animal, it cannot cause a full-strength attack of the disease. This was a major breakthrough for medical science. Not only was the germ theory of disease proven by these experiments, but Pasteur was also bringing humanity closer to the ability to effectively fight deadly sicknesses. He also found a way to

THEY MADE HISTORY: LOUIS PASTEUR

Louis Pasteur was born on December 27, 1822, in Dôle, France. Pasteur worked hard at school but was not remembered as an especially gifted student. He went on to receive his doctor of science degree in 1847 and married Marie Laurent two years later. They had five children, though just two survived to become adults.

In 1854, Pasteur became a professor of chemistry at the University of Lille. During his time there, he learned that germs cause fermentation, putrefaction (decay), infection, and souring. His studies led to the process of pasteurization, which makes food like milk safer by destroying the bacteria that spoils it. He then turned his focus to germ theory.

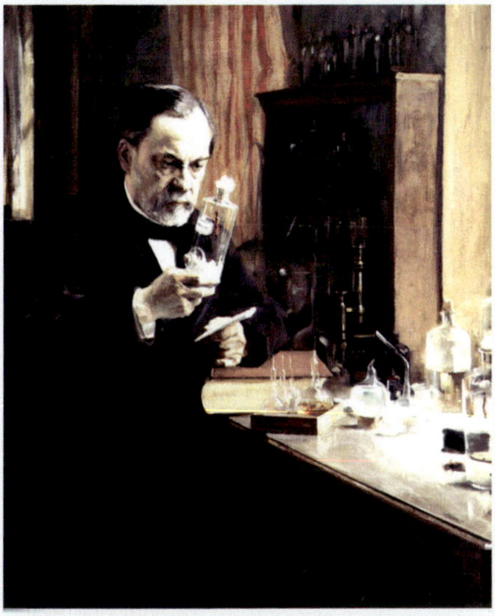

In this oil painting from around 1889, French scientist Louis Pasteur does research in his laboratory.

In 1868, Pasteur became partly paralyzed and could not leave his bed for months. However, he did recover and went on to focus his work on the development of vaccines. Without a doubt, Pasteur's work saved countless people and continues to save lives. He died on September 28, 1895.

HISTORY HAPPENED HERE: THE PASTEUR MUSEUM

The Pasteur Museum in Paris, France, honors the life and achievements of scientist Louis Pasteur. The museum includes three main sections. The first is a display of Pasteur's lab equipment—more than 1,000 objects. These are the same items that helped him prove germ theory and develop vaccines. His scientific notebooks are also on exhibit. Next, visitors are invited to the apartment that the Pasteur family shared from 1888 to 1895. It looks just as it did when they lived there and includes many pieces of art. Finally, below the museum is a mausoleum (tomb) containing the crypt in which Pasteur and his wife are buried.

The museum is located within the Institut Pasteur, the research institute named for Louis Pasteur that has been a home for infectious disease study and other research since 1887. The institute contains more than 130 laboratories and a teaching center dedicated to the same principles that guided Pasteur in his work.

consistently weaken the groups of lethal bacteria by exposing them to extreme heat.

Pasteur used the techniques he learned from cholera to develop a vaccine, or an inoculation of weakened disease bacteria, for another common disease: anthrax. The vaccine was meant to stimulate the body's immune system so that it was better prepared to fight off the disease. Other scientists pushed Pasteur to do a demonstration to publicly prove his theory. On May 5, 1881, with both scientists and newspaper reporters watching, Pasteur and his assistants injected 25 sheep with an anthrax vaccine while 25 other sheep received no vaccine. The next step was to give the vaccinated sheep a few weeks to build up immunity. Then, on May 31, Pasteur injected all 50 sheep with full-strength anthrax germs.

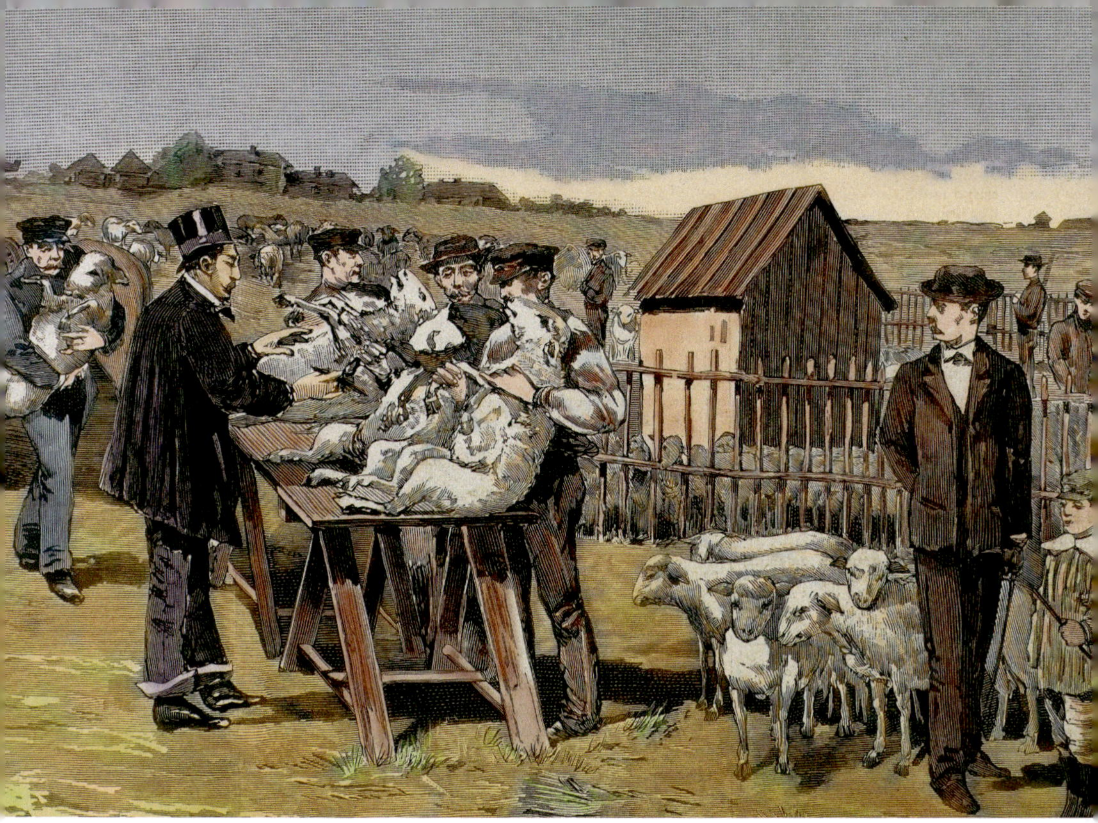

In this engraving, Pasteur inoculates sheep in an attempt to prove that the anthrax vaccine helps build immunity against anthrax.

Many people, including Pasteur's critics, were unsure of what to expect from this new science. However, on June 2, nearly all of the unvaccinated sheep died of anthrax, while all of the vaccinated ones remained healthy. Pasteur had shown clearly that anthrax bacteria caused the disease and, further, that a vaccine made from the same bacteria could make an animal immune to anthrax.

Scientists all across the world were inspired by Pasteur's revolutionary experiment, and they began isolating and studying the germs that cause a number of harmful diseases. One of Pasteur's associates, Alexandre Yersin, isolated the bubonic plague bacterium now bearing his name—*Yersinia pestis*—in 1894. (A Japanese scientist named Kitasato Shibasaburo also discovered the bacterium around the same time as Yersin, after an outbreak of plague in China.) Yersin also tried to discover the ways that the disease

FROM THE SOURCE: SIMOND'S EXPERIMENT

French scientist Paul-Louis Simond, who established that the Oriental rat flea was the main carrier of bubonic plague, later recalled his excitement when his experiment was successful in confirming his suspicions:

> *Without delay I proceeded to the experiment I had in mind ... I had discovered Yersin's bacillus in the digestive tract of fleas taken from plague-ridden rats ... I was fortunate enough to catch a plague infected rat in the home of a plague victim. In the rat's fur there were several fleas running around ...*
>
> *That day, 2 June 1898, I felt an emotion that was inexpressible in the face of the thought that I had uncovered a secret that had tortured man since the appearance of plague in the world. The mechanism of the propagation [spread] of plague includes the transporting of the microbe by rat and man, its transmission from rat to rat, from human to human, from rat to human and from human to rat by parasites [fleas].*[1]

1. Quoted in Marc Simond, et al., "Paul-Louis Simond and His Discovery of Plague Transmission by Rat Fleas: A Centenary," *Journal of the Royal Society of Medicine*, February 1998, p. 102.

was transferred to humans but was unable to confirm any. Not long afterward, French scientist Paul-Louis Simond, who worked at the Institut Pasteur in Paris, found that the main carrier of the deadly plague was the Oriental rat flea.

Thanks in large part to scientists such as Pasteur, Yersin, Kitasato, Simond, and other modern medical researchers, plague no longer causes the misery and death it did in past centuries. A plague vaccine now exists and is effective for all but a small percentage of people. It is made of *Yersinia pestis* that has been

PAST MEETS PRESENT: PLAGUE TODAY

Although it is unusual to develop plague today, it is not impossible. In the United States, about seven people are treated for plague each year on average. Canada has not had a case since 1939. Worldwide, about 2,000 people contract plague annually, mostly in the Democratic Republic of the Congo, Madagascar, and Peru.

Contact with infected fleas remains the cause of plague spread, so experts recommend wearing long pants, socks, and bug repellant when outside, avoiding sick or dead animals, and keeping pets on leashes in areas where plague has occurred. However, if someone contracts plague, antibiotics—often taken for seven to fourteen days—can usually successfully rid the body of the harmful bacteria causing the illness. It is also recommended that those with plague be quarantined to prevent possible spread.

In 2002, a couple from Santa Fe, New Mexico, were bitten by plague-carrying fleas in their own backyard. Though the wife recovered quickly, her husband developed septicemic plague—the most lethal form of the disease. In the 14th century, septicemic plague had a death rate of nearly 100 percent. However, thanks to modern medicine, the husband survived.

In 2015, two people—a teenager and an adult—contracted plague in different parts of Colorado. Unfortunately, the symptoms of the disease were not recognized in time and both died.

In 2018, a young boy in Idaho contracted bubonic plague, the first case of plague in that state in 26 years. Antibiotics successfully helped the child recover. It was not certain where he had contracted the disease. However, squirrels near his home had tested positive a few years before, a reminder that plague's animal reservoirs may spill over into the human population at any time.

inactivated by the chemical formaldehyde. However, doctors say it is only necessary for people who live or work in areas where plague is known to exist to get vaccinated. Still, it is paramount for people everywhere to remember that the disease still exists and to contact medical professionals for help if they suspect they have any symptoms. Incidents of plague still occur from time to time.

"The Nastiest Thing Alive"

Scientist and professor Olaf Schneewind asserted, "*Yersinia pestis* is the nastiest thing alive. It's the most virulent bacterial organism known to mankind."[3] This is why the plague bacterium continues to be a subject of interest to both scientists and historians.

It may seem impossible to have a reoccurrence of widespread disease at the magnitude of the Black Death. However, experts continually warn that we should realize that our society has limitations, even with medical advances. The worldwide COVID-19 outbreak, which began in 2019, showed that a wave of frightening disease could come from anywhere and quickly spread because of how globally connected modern society is.

Even a disease we think we have figured out, like plague, presents difficulties. In fact, the World Health Organization (WHO) categorized plague as a "re-emerging" disease in the late 1990s because of the rising number of cases around the world. Some even think that the bacterium could be weaponized, that is, used as a weapon by warring nations. Luckily, scientists have figured out exactly how the bacterium attacks the body, paving the way for an even more effective vaccine.

American historian William H. McNeill discussed how diseases should be studied as part of history, noting how they can change humankind's place in the balance of nature: "No one can doubt that the role of infectious diseases in the natural balance has been and remains of key importance."[4] Researchers—such as those at the Institut Pasteur of France and the National Institute of Allergy and Infectious Diseases in the United States—are always at work to battle diseases and medical mysteries. These experts are able to collaborate with each other to work together to find solutions, thanks to modern technology. The global toll of the COVID-19 pandemic, which killed millions in a little more than a year, and the race to find an effective vaccine against it have demonstrated that understanding diseases and their impact on society is as critical today as ever to ensure the survival of the human race.

How You See History

1. What kinds of lessons can people today learn from the story of the Black Death and the plague epidemics that followed?
2. Do any facts or stories about the Black Death feel particularly relevant to life in the age of COVID-19?
3. Why are people today still fascinated by the Black Death?

TIMELINE

1330s

Plague emerges in central Asia and moves west, possibly through the fur trade.

1346

As Mongols lay siege to Kaffa, a town on the Crimean peninsula, they catapult plague-infected bodies over the walls.

1347

The Black Death arrives in Constantinople, Sicily, Italy, and France.

1348

The Black Death reaches England as well as parts of the Persian Empire, Greece, Bulgaria, Romania, Poland, and Egypt. Massacres of Jewish communities begin in France. Flagellants begin their movement in Germany.

1349

Plague spreads to Scotland, Wales, Ireland, and Scandinavia.

1350

Eastern Europe is infected by plague.

1351

Plague begins to die out in many parts of Europe.

1361

A new outbreak of plague strikes parts of Europe, particularly affecting children.

1405–1406

England suffers from its first major outbreak of plague in the 15th century.

1665–1666

An unexpected outbreak of plague kills tens of thousands of London's inhabitants.

1894

As an outbreak of plague occurs in China, Swiss scientist Alexandre Yersin identifies the bacterium that causes the disease. Japanese scientist Kitasato Shibasaburo confirms this finding within days of Yersin's discovery.

1897

Development of the first plague vaccine begins.

1900–1904

Bubonic plague strikes the U.S. city of San Francisco, California, where it kills 122 people.

2011

Scientists identify a strain of *Yersinia pestis* in the teeth of Black Death victims at the East Smithfield cemetery in London, England, confirming it was the source of the Black Death but different from the strain that exists today.

2017

A plague outbreak in Madagascar occurs, with more than 2,000 people contracting the disease and more than 200 dying of it.

NOTES

Introduction: A Horrible Chapter in History

1. Giovanni Boccaccio, *Decameron*, trans. J. G. Nichols (New York, NY: Knopf, 2009), p. 10.
2. Boccaccio, p. 8.
3. Thucydides, *History of the Peloponnesian War*, trans. Rex Warner (New York, NY: Penguin, 1972), pp. 152–153.
4. Procopius, *History of the Wars*, trans. H. B. Dewing (Cambridge, MA: Harvard University Press, 1935), pp. 457–458.
5. Procopius, pp. 451–452.

Chapter One: The Black Death Begins

1. Quoted in Rosemary Horrox, *The Black Death* (Manchester, UK: Manchester University Press, 1994), p. 17.
2. Quoted in Johannes Nohl, *The Black Death: A Chronicle of the Plague*, trans. C. H. Clarke (Yardley, PA: Westholme, 2006), pp. 18–19.
3. Quoted in Nohl, p. 18.
4. Giovanni Boccaccio, *Decameron*, trans. J. G. Nichols (New York, NY: Knopf, 2009), p. 12.
5. Boccaccio, pp. 12–13.
6. Quoted in A. R. Myers, ed., *English Historical Documents 1327–1485* (Gloucestershire, UK: Routledge, 1996), p. 88.
7. Quoted in Otto Friedrich, *The End of the World: A History* (New York, NY: Fromm International, 1994), p. 125.

Chapter Two: The Public Panics

1. Quoted in Rosemary Horrox, *The Black Death* (Manchester, UK: Manchester University Press, 1994), pp. 160–161.
2. Barbara W. Tuchman, *A Distant Mirror: The Calamitous 14th Century* (New York, NY: Ballantine, 1996), p. 109.
3. James C. Giblin, *When Plague Strikes: The Black Death, Smallpox, AIDS* (New York, NY: HarperCollins, 1997), pp. 32–33.

4. Quoted in Paul Halsall, ed., "Jewish History Sourcebook: The Black Death and the Jews 1348–1349 CE," Internet History Sourcebooks Project, www.fordham.edu/halsall/jewish/1348-jewsblackdeath.html (accessed May 11, 2020).
5. Quoted in Philip Ziegler, *The Black Death* (New York, NY: Harper Perennial, 2009), p. 5.
6. Otto Friedrich, *The End of the World: A History* (New York, NY: Fromm International, 1994), p. 134.

Chapter Three: Finding the Cause

1. David Herlihy, *The Black Death and the Transformation of the West*, ed. Samuel K. Cohn Jr. (Cambridge, MA: Harvard University Press, 1997), pp. 20–21.
2. James C. Giblin, *When Plague Strikes: The Black Death, Smallpox, AIDS* (New York, NY: HarperCollins, 1997), p. 14.
3. Giblin, pp. 11–12.
4. Philip Ziegler, *The Black Death* (New York, NY: Harper Perennial, 2009), p. 18.

Chapter Four: A Shift in Society

1. Robert S. Gottfried, *The Black Death: Natural and Human Disaster in Medieval Europe* (New York, NY: The Free Press, 1985), p. 94.
2. Matteo Villani, *Universal Chronicle*, excerpted in Perry M. Rogers, *Aspects of Western Civilization* (Upper Saddle River, NJ: Prentice Hall, 2000), pp. 353–365.
3. David Herlihy, *The Black Death and the Transformation of the West*, ed. Samuel K. Cohn Jr. (Cambridge, MA: Harvard University Press, 1997), p. 47.
4. Philip Ziegler, *The Black Death* (New York, NY: Harper Perennial, 2009), p. 247.
5. Quoted in Paul Halsall, ed., "Medieval Source Book: Jean Froissart: On the Jacquerie, 1358," Internet History Sourcebooks Project, sourcebooks.fordham.edu/halsall/source/froissart2.asp (accessed May 11, 2020).

Chapter Five: Cultural Consequences

1. Jean de Venette, *The Chronicle of Jean de Venette*, trans. Jean Birdsall (New York, NY: Columbia University Press, 1953), p. 51.
2. Philip Ziegler, *The Black Death* (New York, NY: Harper Perennial, 2009), p. 279.
3. James C. Giblin, *When Plague Strikes: The Black Death, Smallpox, AIDS* (New York, NY: HarperCollins, 1997), p. 43.
4. David Herlihy, *The Black Death and the Transformation of the West*, ed. Samuel K. Cohn Jr. (Cambridge, MA: Harvard University Press, 1997), pp. 49–50.
5. William H. McNeill, *Plagues and Peoples* (New York, NY: Anchor, 1998), p. 193.

Chapter Six: The Reappearing Plague

1. Robert S. Gottfried, *The Black Death: Natural and Human Disaster in Medieval Europe* (New York, NY: Macmillan, 1985), p. 130.
2. Quoted in John Fenn, *Paston Letters: Original Letters Written During the Reigns of Henry VI, Edward the IV, and Richard III*, vol. 1. (London, UK: Charles Knight, 1840), p. 63.
3. Quoted in "Studies Reveal How Plague Disables Immune System, and How to Exploit the Process to Make a Vaccine," The University of Chicago Medical Center, July 27, 2005, www.uchicagomedicine.org/forefront/news/studies-reveal-howplague-disables-immune-system-and-how-to-exploit-the-process-to-make-a-vaccine.
4. William H. McNeill, *Plagues and Peoples* (New York, NY: Anchor, 1998), p. 23.

FOR MORE INFORMATION

Books: Nonfiction

Cantor, Norman F. *In the Wake of the Plague: The Black Death and the World It Made*. New York, NY: Simon & Schuster Paperbacks, 2015.

Green, Monica H., ed. *Pandemic Disease in the Medieval World: Rethinking the Black Death*. York, UK: Arc Humanities Press, 2015.

Jeffrey, Gary. *The Black Death*. New York, NY: Crabtree Publishing, 2015.

Krasner, Barbara. *Bubonic Plague: How the Black Death Changed History*. North Mankato, MN: Capstone Press, 2019.

Snowden, Frank M. *Epidemics and Society: From the Black Death to the Present*. New Haven, CT: Yale University Press, 2020.

Books: Fiction

Boccaccio, Giovanni. *Decameron*. Translated by John Payne. Hollywood, FL: Simon & Brown, 2018.

Camus, Albert. *The Plague*. New York, NY: Penguin Books, 2020.

Jones, Rob Lloyd. *The Black Death*. London, UK: Usborne Publishing Ltd., 2018.

Websites

Black Death

www.ancient.eu/Black_Death/

The Ancient History Encyclopedia offers an up-to-date overview of the Black Death and its aftermath.

The Black Death

www.bbc.co.uk/bitesize/guides/z7r7hyc/revision/1

The BBC's "bite size" pieces of information about the Black Death make the subject easier to comprehend.

Black Death

www.dkfindout.com/us/history/black-death/

DK Publishing provides information about the Black Death, including a map of where and when it spread.

The Black Death, 1348

www.eyewitnesstohistory.com/plague.htm

This site uses firsthand information from Italian writer Giovanni Boccaccio to inform readers about how people in the 14th century understood plague and its effects on society.

What Was the Black Death?

www.livescience.com/what-was-the-black-death.html

Crucial questions and answers about plague and its impact are answered here.

INDEX

PHOTO CREDITS

Cover ariy/Shutterstock.com; pp. 4, 49, 73 Hulton Archive/Stringer/Hulton Archive/Getty Images; pp. 7, 26, 45, 51 PHAS/Contributor/Universal Images Group/Getty Images; p. 8 Bettmann/Contributor/Bettmann/Getty Images; p. 9 Fine Art/Contributor/Corbis Historical/Getty Images; p. 10 David Spears FRPS FRMS/Corbis Documentary/Getty Images; p. 17 Stock Montage/Contributor/Archive Photos/Getty Images; p. 18 DEA Picture Library/Contributor/De Agostini/Getty Images; p. 19 Science & Society Picture Library/Contributor/SSPL/Getty Images; p. 20 Fourleaflover/iStock/Getty Images Plus/Getty Images; p. 21 MOLA/Contributor/Hulton Archive/Getty Images; p. 24 Dan Kitwood/Staff/Getty Images News/Getty Images; pp. 27, 55 Heritage Images/Contributor/Hulton Fine Art Collection/Getty Images; pp. 32, 57 Heritage Images/Contributor/Hulton Archive/Getty Images; pp. 35, 64 Print Collector/Contributor/Hulton Archive/Getty Images; p. 38 Smith Collection/Gado/Contributor/Archive Photos/Getty Images; p. 43 Courtesy of the CDC; p. 47 CDC/ Dr. Jack Poland; p. 52 Culture Club/Contributor/Hulton Archive/Getty Images; pp. 61, 77, 80 Universal History Archive/Contributor/Universal Images Group/Getty Images; p. 63 Photo Josse/Leemage/Contributor/Corbis Historical/Getty Images; p. 66 Bildagentur-online/Contributor/Universal Images Group/Getty Images; p. 69 DEA/A. Dagli Orti/Contributor/De Agostini/Getty Images; p. 71 Education Images/Contributor/Universal Images Group/Getty Images; p. 83 Christophel Fine Art/Contributor/Universal Images Group/Getty Images; pp. 85, 87 UniversalImagesGroup/Contributor/Universal Images Group/Getty Images.

ABOUT THE AUTHOR

Therese Harasymiw has written and edited more than 200 nonfiction books for children and teens, including books on bacteria, viruses, and plague. Harasymiw received an English degree from Providence College and a master of education degree in English education from the State University of New York at Buffalo. A former high school literature teacher, she works as an editor in educational publishing. Harasymiw, her husband, and their two sons reside in Rochester, New York.